Motives, emotions & memory – exploring how doctors think

Selected posts from the *Illusions of Autonomy* blog

By Philip Berry MD MRCP

Cover symbols

Cardiac arrest, ventricular fibrillation

Morpheus, the God of dreams or sleep, representing palliative care

Chi-Ro, an early Christogram, representing the spiritual heterogeneity of patients and doctors

Daily Mail headline, representing the Liverpool Care Pathway controversy

Butterfly, representing the scheme to improve awareness and care of dementia sufferers

Hyperlinks

Underlined words and sentences are hyperlinks to free sources on the internet; you will need to access the blog in order to find your way to these.

Blog

www.illusionsofautonomy.wordpress.com

Discover other books by this author at Amazon.com

Introduction

I wrote these blog posts to explain the words and actions of doctors in ethically challenging situations. It was a cheeky thing to attempt, as I could not pretend to speak for others in presenting the results of my own reflections. However, feedback from medical and non-medical readers alike soon confirmed that the descriptions reflected their own experiences, which came as a huge relief.

The posts fall into eight categories, but they have a common theme - a desire to explore how doctors balance their human qualities and frailties with what is expected of them. I focus on the way normal men and women react. How do they maintain compassion and reason despite repeated exposure to the misfortune of others? How do they move between emotionally intense scenes without allowing the impact of the first to colour the outcome of the second? How do they discuss end of life care sensitively when time is short and the right thing seems '*so obvious*'? How, on a bad day, do they make patients feel central in their thoughts…when their thoughts are miles away?

One method is to take the essence of a real situation (drawn from my years of experience as a hospital doctor) and to enlarge it, dissect it, using imaginary dialogue. Another is to make a quick survey of the literature, or to examine a particularly hard case known to all in the media. In one post I analyse the evidence given in the Court of Protection ('Quality of life projections: do doctors have any idea?'). In 'A Never Event and the chain of blame' I construct a completely fictional set of lethal circumstances. Throughout, care is been taken to dissociate fictional patients from those who were involved in the historical scenario that stimulated the essay. Confidentiality is never compromised.

Decisions taken with patients towards the end of life are developed within the framework of 'Good Medical Practise' (GMP), a series of guidelines published by the GMC. If all decisions adhered to GMP there would be no controversy. Every management plan would result from mutual understanding between patient and doctor. Their goals, their understanding of risk, burden and benefit, their fully informed consent to treatment, would be ascertained well in advance. If they lacked mental capacity, those factors would be agreed by those who knew them best. If only it were that straightforward! Many of these blog posts were generated by my reflections on scenarios that did not fit easily into that scheme; situations in which major decisions about life extending treatment had to be made quickly, in the absence of background information, in isolation from patents' representatives... At times like these accusations of paternalism can arise; and autonomy becomes just an illusion. The good intentions of doctors making those decisions have to be presumed, and the sensible application of their years of experience respected.

Something happened in 2012 to undermine that presumption of goodness - the Liverpool Care Pathway controversy. It was my horrified reaction to accusations of immorality and systemic euthanasia, as they multiplied in the press, that spurred me to begin writing. I could see trust in my profession eroding…unjustifiably (in my opinion). The LCP furore appears to have died down now, but other scandals, such as wrongdoing at Mid-Staffordshire, or alleged cover-ups at the Care Quality Commission, have compounded the damage. There is much rebuilding to do. Perhaps, by being open and honest about the way doctors handle ethically complex situations, these posts can contribute in a small way to that recovery.

I am hugely grateful to the support of readers, especially those I have found via Twitter. Their positive feedback has kept me motivated.

London, June 2013
@philaberry

Part 1: The psychology of doctors

The Onion Cellar: crying at work, crying at home

Have you cried at work? Do you show the depth of your emotions when faced with tragic clinical circumstances? I have never cried, and it is unusual for clinical situations to even moisten my eyes. Although I have been tempted to hug patients when they appear emotionally broken, I am far too inhibited to break through that force-field of unfamiliarity. A gentle hand on the shoulder or leg is about as intimate as it gets really.

This is not true for all doctors – some are much more comfortable with displays of sympathy or warmth...but we are all different. How do we describe doctors who admit to being moved to tears? Sentimental? A sentimental person is predisposed to be moved or swayed by emotions; it is a normal characteristic, but one that is repressed to a greater or lesser extent in most working lives. The *empathetic* doctor on the other hand will feel sadness and grief when they see their patients cursed by nature's caprice, and will allow this to inform their own understanding. The *sentimental* doctor will reflect and display those emotions, and be visibly affected. If we accept that a continuum exists which encompasses these two characteristics, knowing where, or how, to draw the line is a huge challenge. Particular circumstances may pull individual doctors over that line now and again. When that happens, we cry. This tendency must be balanced with cool professionalism, for if sentimentality reigns there may be a deficiency of dispassionate thought.

So what lies at the other end of that continuum? How do we describe those who appear to feel no emotion at all? Does their stony facade hide inner turmoil? Are they likely to suffer from a build up unresolved mini-traumas? Or can they function indefinitely without releasing those emotions? Well, perhaps the key word here is 'appear'. We can only know as much as we can see, and the profundity of their feeling may well be hidden from us.

In 'To Cry or Not to Cry: Physicians and Emotions at the Bedside' by Navneet Majhail and Erica Warlick, an account is given of a bone marrow transplant physician who cried when a young patient whom she knew well discussed the likelihood of death.

All agreed that she would not want to continue with aggressive measures and allowing her to die peacefully would be in her best interest. At an emotionally intense moment, her primary BMT physician's eyes began to water, and she shed a few tears prior to regaining composure and continuing the conversation. As the team left the room, the medical student asked, "Is it OK to cry in front of a patient?"

In response to this an <u>informal survey of other physicians'</u> <u>attitudes</u> to the display of emotion was undertaken. The selection of responses is fascinating, and very measured. For instance:

"I think that it is totally fine not to cry ... If that is not in your nature ... a physician should express some genuine sympathy/empathy for a grieving family, but it can be done with words or mannerisms."

"I think it is a problem if the emotional moment is primarily about the physician's feelings ... But if the context is about the patient or the family's feelings then I think it is good to show empathy. ... If the "primary gain" is to make the family or patient feel better ... then it is OK ... whereas if the primary gain is to make the physician feel better ... then that is not OK."

"I think it is acceptable to break down the austerity of the medical relationship at times ... when families and patients need someone they trust the most (e.g., end of- life crisis), the emotion we show only helps bridge the divide that we've built within medicine."

And this one reflected my own thoughts very closely:

"There can be a fine line between being compassionate and empathetic versus allowing emotions to adversely cloud recommendations for patient care."

A 2008 New York Times article by Barron H. Lerner explored the question 'At Bedside, Stay Stoic or Display Emotions?' He (and the fact that he is a 'he' becomes relevant) contrasts the behaviour of two physicians. There is Dr Benita Burke, who was in the habit of,

'...skipping lunch to spend extra time with her cancer patients. They dubbed this time 'mental health rounds,' during which they could address issues that were not strictly medical. Many times, Dr. Burke would wind up in tears or giving an embrace.'

I find that behaviour remarkable – in fact I find it uncomfortably eccentric. In contrast, according to the article, Dr. Hiram S. Cody (acting chief of the breast cancer service at Memorial Sloan-Kettering Cancer Center) adjures his staff,

'to understand, to sympathise, to empathize and to reassure...not to be emotional and/or cry with my patients.' The writer of the article then comments, 'whether because of my personality or my being a man, I, too, have never cried in front of a patient.' (Phew. I am not the only unfeeling man out there!)

In 2006 I wrote an article called 'The Absence of Sadness: Darker Reflections on the Doctor-Patient Relationship', which began with a paradox – recognition that I felt sadder when patients whom I barely knew died, rather than those I had watched suffering for days or weeks on the ward. I was moved (moist eyes, nothing more) by the love shown to a dying man by his family:

'In this case my sadness derived not from torn attachment, but the juxtaposition of familial devotion with death. The brief sketch of his life, drawn during our first interaction in casualty, contained only positive images. My appreciation of him as a person was unchallenged, our relationship unsullied by the more complicated emotions that can accumulate on the ward.'

Then, having described various threats to the patient-physician relationship, I conclude,

'The tensions created by sudden, severe or incurable illness settle on the most vulnerable aspect of our experience with patients; not our medical proficiency, not our energy, not our commitment to advocacy...but our sense of attachment.'

So, if emotion cannot be explored (by some of us) at work, where can it be resolved? I have read some very emotional medical accounts recently. One example is Elin Lowri's beautiful blog post about the importance of love in the inevitable progress of death. A number of commentators have admitted that they were moved tears. I certainly felt emotional, and that is saying a lot, for me! I asked myself how it is that someone like me can be moved by such well-written words at home, while being in little danger of sniffing back tears in the workplace. Then I was reminded of the *Onion Cellar.*

In The Tin Drum, by Gunter Grass, people who have been deprived of the opportunity to display emotion pay good money to meet in an onion cellar.

> *"...It was this drought, this tearlessness that brought those who could afford it to Schmuh's Onion Cellar, where the host handed them a little cutting board – pig or fish – a paring knife for eighty pfennigs, and for twelve marks an ordinary, field-, garden-, and kitchen-variety onion, and induced them to cut their onions smaller and smaller until the juice – what did the onion juice do? It did what the world and the sorrows of the world could not do: it brought forth a round, human tear. It made them cry. At last they were able to cry again. To cry properly, without restraint, to cry like mad. The tears flowed and washed everything away."*

I wondered, thinking about the right place and the right time for displays of emotion, whether a sentimental reaction to accounts of patients and their illnesses, read outside the workplace and in relation to people that we have never seen, may provide that access of emotion that we cannot readily, or safely, tap into on the awards. Perhaps there is a place for vicarious emotions, whereby the feelings that we probably should be feeling on the wards, as normal, feeling men and women, can be experienced in abstract, at a distance, through the words of others. So please keep those blog posts and articles coming…they are healthy!

Disappearing doctors: the limits of medical debate on Twitter

My adoption of Twitter coincided with the Liverpool Care Pathway (LCP) controversy. Naturally, I 'joined the conversation'. The compact exchanges that followed forced me to examine and re-evaluate my views. The links to press stories (in newspapers I would not normally read) and blogs helped me appreciate how broad the spectrum of opinion is. The cases described in the media are enough to open anyone's eyes to the risks, but the additional voices on Twitter, their views expressed vehemently at times, reinforced the fact that many more have witnessed, or at least perceived, poor practice. I am happier now to accept that the Pathway has not been used well universally, and perhaps, even though the pathway is intrinsically helpful, it needs to be changed to ensure better application. Nevertheless, because I have seen the benefits of the pathway, I have argued forcefully in its favour.

Engaging in the argument demands patience and moderation, because Tweets can be provocative. Accusations of murder are common, and for some this forms the backbone of their case against the LCP. It soon becomes clear when your interlocutor's mind cannot be changed. The intensity rises, the argument gets personal. In some cases it becomes clear that the individual in question had a relative who died in difficult circumstances. Trust in the medical profession and the way it manages end of life care was damaged, and when things go wrong so close to home that damage tends to be irrevocable. Whatever the evidence, however overwhelming the number of voices in favour of the pathway, you are unlikely to overturn the misgivings of someone who has vivid memories of a relative dying in hospital.

Nevertheless, it seems reasonable to continue to argue, for Twitter is a place that gives you time to compose your arguments, and time to digest the points made by others. But here the difficulties arise. As doctors we are trained to sympathise and empathise with the relatives. When we talk with a relative of a dying patient we try to inhabit their point of view and understand what they are saying. If they are angry, we absorb that emotion. If they accuse us, or the hospital, or the system, of making mistakes, we do not challenge them; it's not the right time. These are universal qualities of course, not restricted to doctors, but they are qualities that we have actively developed as part of our vocation.

This is why I find it difficult to maintain opposition to someone whose views are so clearly coloured by personal experience. In trying to overturn their doubts I fear that I am actually belittling their memories of a loved one. So, just as I would never allow myself to become involved in an argument with a patient's relative on the ward, however much I disagreed with them, I am increasingly reluctant to have arguments with those who wish to banish the pathway. The same applies to those affected by poor care at Mid-Staffordshire, or relatives touched by medical error elsewhere. Doctors seem wary of challenging the validity of HSMR statistics, knowing perhaps that Tweets may be read by families involved. It seems impolite. Does this reticence lead to a stifled, incomplete debate?

Perhaps doctors are too ready to adopt a 'customer is always right' approach. We often find ourselves speaking with people, be they patients or relatives, who challenge us. But we absorb the emotion, the occasional animus, the very rare invective; we step back, give it space, let it mellow with time. You can't do that on Twitter, it's about the here and now. And it's loud. When doctors find themselves losing their rag, raising their voice, making it up as they go along, they tend to remove themselves from the scene. They disappear.

The evolution of authority: confidence *vs* arrogance

The journey from timid trainee to clinical leader is rarely a smooth one, and authority does not come easily to all. Lessons learnt from inevitable missteps can be as useful as the positive accumulation of knowledge and skills. By looking back at formative moments in a fourteen year career I have tracked the evolution of my own authority…and in doing so I have recognised that near the end of the path lies a trap, and it is called arrogance.

As a Senior House Officer, in conversation with my Registrar.
Registrar: "And you think the bronchospasm is what, pulmonary eosinophilia, due to migration of parasites? Why doesn't he just have asthma?"
Me: "It's just…this patient has made no improvement after five days. We're getting nowhere. His renal function is off. Either an unusual infection, or something else…perhaps autoimmune, vasculitic. Shall I ask the rheumatologists to see him?"
R: "He's a bit dry, that's all. Speed up the fluids and his kidneys will turn around. The prednisone will kick in soon. Don't worry."

Next day – a SHO detains me in the corridor
SHO: "I hear your man was transferred to intensive care."

Me: "I've seen him. Blew a pupil, dropped his conscious level. I don't understand, it doesn't add up."

SHO: "But you've heard what the diagnosis is?"

Me: "No. Not yet. Tell me."

SHO: "Churg-Strauss syndrome. Classic presentation. ICU called the rheumatologists in. But he's pretty far gone now, on dialysis…they're starting cyclophosphamide this afternoon. You look shocked."

A few years later, with some specialised knowledge under my belt, I felt confident in challenging error where I saw it developing…

In the intensive care unit, a Specialist Trainee greets me.

ST: "Thanks for coming down. Her liver is fine but her ammonia is off the scale. Very odd. Epileptic, but the EEG says she's not in status. CT scan is normal"

Me: "Does she take valproate? An overdose would explain it – it interrupts the urea cycle."

ST: "Yes. We figured that. But she hasn't woken up on the filter. Have you got any ideas?"

Me: "I've had a look at her. She has signs of raised intracranial pressure. Clonus, sluggish pupils. She's at risk of coning. At the moment you have no handle on the pressure, nor how aggressively to treat it. She needs a bolt."

ST: "An intracranial pressure monitor? Really?"

Me: "Yes, the neurosurgeons will put one in if you call them."

Later that day

Me: "Did the neurosurgeons come down?"

ST: "No. We didn't think it would add much."

Me: "But it would…you have no idea what's going on in her skull."

ST: "But the treatment would be the same anyway. And besides, there's no evidence of a survival advantage…"

Me: "Evidence is lacking, you're right. But this situation is rare, the trials will never be done. Look, you asked for my advice, and I've given it to you."

ST: "We're not convinced…it's a risky intervention…"

How far do I take this? I'm convinced it's the right thing to do. How hard should I fight for what (I think) I know is the right decision?

Me: "This woman is at huge risk of brain death, and without quantitative assessment of the pressure you cannot treat her appropriately. If the pressure is persistently high after mannitol you'll need to try indomethacin, consider a thiopentone induced coma, cool her right down. Where's your consultant? Who do I need to convince to make this happen? You clearly don't have the experience in this unit to make the right decision."

But I did not say that. I figured – *it's their decision, their responsibility in the end. I gave an opinion, one of many probably,*

and they must assess the pro's and con's before making the call.
They may have a better understanding of the whole situation. So I
said,

"I'll review her first thing tomorrow. That will be 24 hours since
she presented. If there are persistent features of raised pressure I
think you'll have to do it. Ask the neurosurgeons for their advice.
You have mine."

She never woke up. No-one can be sure what difference the bolt
would have made.

Two years later I found myself arguing over a patient whose heart
had stopped.

Me: "Another cycle, and then I think we'll stop. There's been no
electrical activity since we started…all agree?"
The cardiology Registrar enters the cubicle pushing a portable
echocardiography machine.
Cardiology Registrar: "I'm just going to take a look, see if there's
any ventricular activity."
Me: "We're just about to call it. She's dead, unfortunately. We've
been going for 20 minutes in asystole."
CR: "You haven't excluded all reversible causes yet. What about
tamponade?"
Me: "There's no reason to suspect tamponade, no instrumentation,
anticoagulation, no electrical activity on the monitor…"

CR: "It will only take a couple of minutes. My consultant will want to know before you stop resuscitation."

Me: "What! No! I'm running this arrest, we've given four shots of adrenaline, and the line is flat. She is dead. I'm not going to have this woman subjected to another 10 minutes of CPR while you do an echo and go and call your consultant."

CR: "It's protocol on the cardiology ward."

Nurse: "That's two minutes."

Me: "Okay, what's the rhythm…asystole, not compatible with a pulse. Let's stop. Stop compressions."

CR: "I'm calling my consultant."

Me: "Do so. At no point in the life support algorithm does it mention echocardiograms and phone calls to consultants. We're stopping."

I walked away, emboldened by the challenge. Assuming authority in this situation had come easily. I felt that I had risen to the challenge, and proved my seniority.

Two weeks into my job as a consultant I conducted a ward round. A new patient, with alcoholic cirrhosis, had been transferred to the ward. My SHO presented him.

"He's been triggering all night, low blood pressure. Down to 80 systolic."

"He's septic you said."

"Yes, spontaneous bacterial peritonitis, confirmed."

"He's passing urine, he looks alert. Lactate's normal. Give him more time, he should skate through without needing vasopressors."

Later that day my SHO found me in endoscopy.

"He's not picking up. We'll need to adjust the alarm parameters if we don't want to be bleeped about his BP every thirty minutes."

"This is
what cirrhotics do, run low BPs, dilated circulations, even without sepsis. A bit more filling, another couple of days of antibiotics and he should turn around."

Next morning she came to my office; the registrar was away.

"I'm worried. Sodium's down, BP is still poor. And he's got a rash, all over his trunk. It's blue."

"But he's talking, reading the paper, walking to the toilet. I passed him on the ward this morning. I'm not too concerned about him."

"But he's just not right…"

A brief stab of annoyance interrupted my continued reassurances – yes, we're all worried about him, but get on with it!

On the third morning I was called to the ICU. My patient lay dying, his skin mottled, a cardiac output monitor confirming that his heart was barely functioning. He had been displaying signs of

25

severe alcoholic cardiomyopathy from day one, and I had missed it. My SHO had never seen a case before, but she had *sensed* it, the wrongness...just as I had sensed that there must be an alternative diagnosis in the man with asthma. I didn't hear her, because I was sure I knew more.

The only doctor we can observe over an entire career is the one we see in the mirror every morning. We must reflect on our own experiences to truly understand how we have evolved – and why. When the patient with Churg-Strauss syndrome was admitted I was no more than a wallflower during medical arguments. Now, if I am sure of myself, and if after reasoned argument I wish to ensure that the wrong decision is not made, I may display intransigence and will ultimately pull rank. For after all, I am right more often than I am wrong, and my senior position should ensure that what I say goes. Shouldn't it?

Having reflected on some of the steps that led from a questioning but silent observer to a physician with the power to insist, I am reminded that the evolution of authority does not end with the progression to consultant rank. Only open mindedness, the ability to admit mistakes (to oneself if not to ones juniors), and the realization that learning occurs in both directions can prevent the sheen of hard earned authority from deteriorating into a impermeable hide of arrogance.

The limits of responsibility

A few months ago I looked after a patient from eastern Europe who presented with episodes of confusion and weakness. He had lost a great deal of weight, and his skin had become pigmented* over the previous four months. His wife, ever present, was highly critical of the care that he received even though we arranged three scans and a lumbar puncture within 48 hours of admission. After five days I raised the possibility of heavy metal toxicity (he was an electrician, they are prone to Manganese poisoning), although the differential diagnosis was very wide. Deliberate arsenic poisoning was on my mind, but it was way down the list. Still, if you don't think about these things you never make the clever diagnosis. That's what I tell my juniors.

Twenty-four hours later his wife arranged overland transfer to his home town in a Baltic state. The two of them just disappeared off the ward. The doctor who received them emailed me, asking for a summary. Two weeks later she sent another message informing me he had died. A post-mortem was refused. The case bugged me. I had a strong desire to travel out there, find the town, walk into the hospital (a grey, functional building in my mind's eye) and demand an exhumation. Or, at the very least, find some tissue, a hair off a brush, an old toe nail, something to analyse. But then, what did this have to do with me? Our local heavy metal expert did not think the clinical features were typical, and really, how on earth could I achieve anything? It was not my concern. House might have jumped on a plane, or sent one of his photogenic protégés, but here was no professional or moral obligation for me to discover the truth. I had reached the limit of my responsibility.

There are other occasions when I find myself trying to define the limits of my responsibility. I have a patient who is alcoholic, cirrhotic… he is likely to die soon if he does not stop drinking. I have referred him to the appropriate agencies, but they require patients to attend of their own volition, to demonstrate an ongoing commitment. He will not. His mother writes to me asking me to sort something out. What can I do? I write to his GP and to the addiction services; I detox him when turns up in the emergency room. But I can't own his alcoholism. As he walks out of the door, temporarily mended, he passes beyond my sphere of influence. That's the limit of my responsibility.

Now imagine this: I travel to that Baltic state and confirm that my patient was poisoned (by his wife?). Justice is done, based on my little hunch. Imagine I admit my alcoholic patient, detoxify him, counsel him, work on him with psychologists and addiction specialists (to hell with 'length of stay' pressures)…until he is freed of his terrible illness. A phenomenal result. The extra mile, the refusal to recognise conventional limits, the difference between adequate and exemplary. Should I?

A more quotidien example. I started a patient on a powerful new medication (Azathioprine) one week before going on holiday. Foolhardy perhaps, but he was keen. I arranged for him to have a blood test a day before his departure, and I promised to tell him if it showed any signs that the tablet was reacting badly with him. But I was away that day and asked my registrar to look them up. She remembered, but at the end of the day, just before heading home. The results were not good. His liver had become acutely inflamed. Referring to the computerised patient information system she found that his phone number was not listed. There was no way of telling him to stop the new medication. She sent me a text – passing the buck back to her boss! I worried about it that evening, and awoke the following morning no more relaxed. I e-mailed my secretary over breakfast, at 6.30 in the morning, asking her to call the GP at 8 am, her first task on arriving at the office. At nine, when I arrived in my off-site clinic, she e-mailed me the patient's phone number. I called. He was walking out of his front door when the phone rang. The taxi was waiting outside his house. Situation salvaged!

On that occasion the limit of responsibility had extended beyond working hours into my mind, where the danger of the situation festered and ensured that I woke with a single mission: to contact him. It's a fairly unremarkable example, but it illustrates how the limits of responsibility enlarge in proportion to the risks that we take as doctors, with our patients. Every junior doctor I know works late. It is habitual, and it makes a mockery of the European Working Time Directive. Nevertheless, shifts are shorter, handovers are more frequent, and it is important that juniors learn to balance the instinct to 'complete' with the reasonable pressure to drop what they are working on, ring a colleague and get home.

So, while learning how to erect professional boundaries, they must also recognise the situations that demand an extra effort. They must identify the problems that will spill over into their leisure time, distract them during the weekend, force them to pick up the phone despite their family's disapproving murmurs, and satisfy themselves that their patient is being looked after properly. Not every week…just now and again.

* Yes, we excluded hypoadrenalism!

Part 2: Compassionate care

Medical relativism: on prioritisation, excuses and kindness

In a recent Clinical Medicine article, '*Doctors and others: reflections on the first Francis Report*' (£) Professor John Saunders writes, 'People do not go into careers in healthcare to be cruel...' and yet, 'many experienced commentators...have witnessed an absence of kindness: an attitudinal change that resulted in substandard care.' How does this happen? How do we explain the spectrum of kindness shown to patients that results in some coming away from hospital impressed by medical staff and some feeling neglected, as though they were a bother or a burden?

The explanation must lie in factors related to medical staff and patients. Patients come as they are of course, and there is little point analysing their characteristics in the quest to understand the spectrum of kindness. So, what of medical staff? They are human, and they vary. Some express kindness better than others, but even the poor ones are nice some of the time. Some respond better to quiet, unassuming patients who appear grateful, while others show their best side to those who are more demanding and articulate. Some engage fully only when they recognise some special factor – a common link, a mutual acquaintance, an especially tragic set of circumstances, or the perception of professional risk. Some doctors warm up only when the disease in question fires their intellect. None of these psychological explanations are defensible…all patients should receive the same amount of kindness. However, for some reason, some patients appear to *deserve* more kindness than others. It is the perception of deservingness that I wish to focus on, especially its root in the unavoidable practise of medical relativism.

I remember working in A&E departments (in the mid 1990's) where waiting rooms teemed with dozing patients and red LED displays routinely flashed << 8 hours >>. By the time patients were seen their agitation had transformed to resignation, crushed by a sense of powerlessness. On the part of the doctors, a 'warzone' mentality seemed to foster a 'Don't complain, you're lucky to get seen…' attitude. In this environment indifferent care could be delivered, or witnessed, but ignored. That was the just the way it was. Kindness did flower, because there were good people, but the pressure on the system did not allow those flowers to cover the ground.

I wonder if the embers of that attitude smoulder in the minds of older doctors (myself included) whose behaviours were patterned by a sense of continuous battle. I certainly feel it rekindle now and again…for instance when a patient complains for reasons that appear unfounded (about a delay, a lack of explanation, an early discharge). I feel sure that they had good care, and find myself thinking, 'What are they on about? We did pretty well by them. It was incredibly busy, there were people on the ward who were far sicker, we were a doctor down...' I have fallen into the trap of medical relativism, making comparisons between one patient's predicament and another's.

We make comparisons between patients every day. It is part of being a responsible doctor. It absolutely necessary to prioritise, to treat the sickest first (and more intensively) while leaving the less unwell for longer. However, patients arriving in emergency departments, or those waiting to speak to medical teams on the ward, are concerned about their own problems. They do not see the complete picture...and why should they? They are anxious and preoccupied. Given this, is it surprising that they begin to feel hard done by if our explanation for their delay in treatment or attention includes a comparison, between their situation and that of another. The nurse answers the bell 30 minutes after it was pressed, to find a soiled patient;

"I'm so sorry, I was just finishing the drug round..."

So it seems the drug round was more important that their comfort. Perhaps it was, who knows? But the patient won't see it that way. Or a family attends the ward to discuss end of life care with the medical registrar, who is ninety minutes late;

"I do apologise, I got held up with a emergency downstairs. I asked the ward sister to let you know...."

So the sick patient in the high dependency unit is more important than the dying patient on the ward, or the family members who gathered together in the relatives room nearly two hours ago, tense, expectant, not knowing what to say. What are the family to think of this?

One simple solution is to avoid making overt comparisons. Some of us may do this already, because it feels like we are making excuses if we go on about our other duties. It doesn't feel completely professional to explain why we are late, or distracted, or less than focussed…because we know that *our* stress isn't *their* concern. The danger in this policy of concealment is that patients see only the instance of neglect, but not the context in which that neglect arose. We may have justified our less than excellent performance by medical relativism, but the patients only see the end result. They develop a sense of *de*-prioritisation, and are not impressed.

I wonder if unchecked relativism might contribute to the kind of rationalisation and dismissal that allowed poor care to thrive at Mid Staffs. For senior hospital doctors whose careers have seen patients progress from timid supplicants to consumers of services with enhanced autonomy (and very different expectations), it is vital that we make a psychological leap – one that should come easily to anyone who has ever had to receive hospital treatment. Patients don't care what the man or woman in the adjacent bed has; they are concerned about their own problems. They must be

35

reassured the solution to those problems is at the centre of your, their doctor's, thoughts, and not being forever shuffled and de-prioritised by the constant influx of more 'deserving' patients.

I started to write this post before the inflammatory word 'warzone' surfaced in the media once again. On May 9th 2013, Dr Cliff Mann, registrar at the College of Emergency Medicine, used it to describe the current situation in UK A&E departments. As the rising pressure in A&E is transmitted to the wards, maintaining an impression of patient centrality, of an importance that is *intrinsic* and not dependent on the needs and demands of those around them, will become harder and harder.

"It was as though I wasn't there": the problem of the invisible patient

The CQC has published the results of its 2012 national in-patient survey. Some aspects of it were picked up by the Independent newspaper on 16th April 2013. One of the observations in the 'Doctors and Nurses' section is that:

There have been improvements in the results for questions asking about doctors and nurses, with the majority of respondents saying that: Doctors (75%, up from 73% in 2011) and nurses (81%, up from 78% in 2011) did not talk in front of them as if they were not there.

What is the explanation for the other 25% who feel that their doctors did talk as though the patient wasn't there?

1) The doctors thought the patient was not listening, or not able to comprehend what was being said...but they were wrong.

The only way to avoid this would be *never* to speak to a third party (usually a colleague, often a relative) over a patient, even if they appear unconscious or severely impaired cognitively. That seems a sensible rule of thumb…but go to any intensive care unit and you will see very open discussions, concerning life and death, just feet away from sedated patients. It happens. Clearly, as medical practitioners, we are prone to falling into the trap of underestimating the degree of cognitive function in patients who appear, externally, to be unengaged with their surroundings.

2) The doctors conducted technical, impenetrable discussions with colleagues without taking in account the patient's bewilderment.

Here I would like to mount a defence of doctors. On a ward round there are several tasks that have to be achieved. Most, but not all, can easily be followed by a non-medically trained person.

- Greeting and introductions
- Ascertainment of the patient's current symptoms, feelings and concerns,
- Confirmation of what has occurred thus far during the admission
- Physical examination if appropriate
- *Review and scrutiny of medical investigation
- *Interpretation of above data
- Agreed plan (in context of patient's goals)
- Communication of that plan to the patient

- *Additionally, there may be opportunities for teaching.

The starred (*) elements may, in my view, evade the patient's full understanding. This is because the language used will contain technical terms, Latin or Greek derived terminology and a cascade of acronyms. I experienced an example of this recently – there was patient with 'the best bronchial breathing you'll ever hear'. I explained to the patient that he had signs of pneumonia, asked him if the FY1 (the most junior doctor) could listen with her stethoscope, and had the following discussion with her and the team:

'What did you hear?'

'Loud breath sounds.'

'How did it compare to the other side?'

'Louder.'

'Just louder?'

'Different.'

'I would say clearer.'

'Yes, it was.'

'And do you know why?'

'The lung is solid…'

'And that's called….?'

'Bronchial breathing'

'Yes! Well done. And then you might look for other signs such as increased vocal resonance, vocal fremitus, signs that the sound waves are being transmitted through solid lung rather than open alveoli…you might see air bronchograms on the chest x-ray…Mike, what was the white cell count and CRP?"

"12.8 and 87."

"Strep antigen, has that been sent…"

"No. But he's on Co-Amox and Clary…"

And it's moved completely out of the patient's sphere of understanding. I look down, aware that we have progressed onto discussing his laboratory results, and treatment…the mini-teaching session has segued into person-specific details, and the patient does not have a clue what we are talking about. If he was asked to comment on a survey he might well say, 'They talked as though I wasn't there!'

How do we avoid this? Vigilance. Being aware that every single word uttered will be heard and reflected upon by the patient. Any unguarded word. Comparisons with other, historical patients

('...you remember the man we saw last week, on intensive care, he had the same signs...) may lead the patient to fear that they will follow the same course. Mentioning a theoretical differential diagnosis ('...this could be tuberculosis, or a tumour can cause compression and distal collapse...') will cause them to dwell on all the terrible possibilities. It's just not possible to talk 'freely', even though there may be a purely medical justification in considering other diseases or treatments.

Two solutions to improving our conduct during those starred sections are:

a) always use non-technical language

b) move away from the patient's bedside.

There are problems with both in my view.

a) efforts to avoid technical terms during conversations with colleagues often result in a pseudo-medical, strained and patronising tone, or in asides that contain semi-interpretations . For instance, '...we mean the lung has gone solid, from the pus in the air-sacs...it's a normal finding, in pneumonia...fremitus, that means the sound vibrations are felt on the skin...'. Many patients would actually appreciate such interpretation, as it provides an insight into their own condition. Within reason I would support it, but, to be honest, it is the student or house office we are trying to teach about physical signs, not the patient. Certainly in communicating the interpretation and plan such non-technical terms *must* be used, but in their right place I think the 'code' that doctors use is necessary.

 b) moving away can be cumbersome. It may also give the wrong impression, that something more grave is being discussed in secret. Afterwards, the team must go back to the bedside, so an additional awkward phase, wherein the team trundles off to the corridor or nurses' station and then trundles back is introduced. To do that with each patient on a 30 patient ward round is probably unfeasible.

We must find a way of making the patient feel involved while having a discussion that they cannot truly be involved in. This is a demanding expectation. Clearly, in 75% of cases, we achieve it. Perhaps it is in those cases where alert and interested patients with complex and subtle problems that seem to require prolonged technical discussion make up the other 25%. In these cases the acronyms and the secret codes go on and on, interspersed with concerned glances back to the increasingly concerned patient in his or her physically inferior position on the bed…followed by a brief, concluding summary that reminds the patient of one of those comedy sketches where a dishonest interpreter transforms a 90 second string of Chinese into a two word English phrase. It's all about sensitivity and empathy in the end.

My take home message would be – Yes, sometimes it is necessary to talk in a way that will not be fully understood, but make sure the patient is forewarned about those portions of the visit, and make sure you check that their degree of comprehension has been addressed with a suitably clear interpretation. And don't leave without checking that their questions and concerns have been dealt with.

Meaning it: acting, (in)sincerity and compassion on the wards

A consultant and her junior sit opposite the daughter of a dying patient. They have entered the relatives' room following an assessment of the patient on the ward round. The elderly lady is clearly succumbing to pneumonia, and the consultant wants to explain why continued efforts to ventilate non-invasively through a mask and monitor intensely in the high dependency unit are probably not the right things to do. The conversation lasts 15 minutes, for the patient's daughter finds it hard to understand why such aggressive approaches to treatment should not continue. But already it has been going on for four days, and the situation is only got worse.

'I'm sorry Mrs Davis, I really think it's time for us to be honest with you, honest with the patient and with ourselves, and to admit that everything we have done, the antibiotics, the blood tests, the mask, have not made a difference. She's getting anxious and distressed, and the truth that we must accept that this pneumonia is too much for her.'

'But she has got through this type of illness before.'

'I think this really is worse. And that was five years ago…her heart and lungs have grown weaker since then. We really

44

are just keeping her going, keeping her alive, artificially really. The chances of her improving are next to zero now.'

'But she improved at the beginning…'

'She did. She tried, we tried, if there was a chance she would have taken it by now. I'm glad we tried as hard as we did, even if there was a 2, 3, 5 percent chance, it was worth it. But now it has become clear…I'm sorry.'

The relative begins to cry. The junior doctor watches as his consultant reaches to the desk for a box of tissues. She puts a hand on the relative's hand, where it rests on the edge of her seat, and she offers one of the tissues. She takes her time, gives enough space for the daughter to gather herself, but then carries on, without being brutal. The relative seems to understand, and agrees. It's not a case of bulldozing her, just allowing her to take in the truth of the situation. The junior doctor watches in some awe, impressed by his consultant's skill, her ability to empathise, to adjust her tone, to choose just the right words. He decides to emulate her, and to develop the skills that he was observed.

They leave relatives' room. The patient's daughter remains there, teary eyed, fiddling with her mobile phone. Consultant and junior walk back to the nurses' station, where the patient's notes lay open.

'You couldn't get me a continuation sheet could you? I need to write it all down, the usual essay! God…the poor thing never had a chance, I don't know why we've carried on so long. Ten years ago she wouldn't have even been offered non-invasive ventilation…we probably use it too much to be honest…'

Her junior is shocked. He gets the paper, places it into the notes, and watches as his boss writes a version of the discussion down. All those fine words…

What has happened here? Did the consultant actually mean what she said. Was she lying? Is she completely two-faced? Or was she just acting – playing the part? And playing it so well! Was she compassionate? Yes, it looks as though she was. So was she lying *and* practising compassionately at the same time? It seems so.

Ups and downs

Any non-medically trained person following a typical ward round in an acute hospital would be shocked at the range of emotions that is displayed and experienced. A ward round involves giving good news to those who are recovering, and the worst imaginable to those diagnosed with terminal disease. There are conversations with relatives regarding end of life care, and delicate explorations of what patients would have wanted in the final days and weeks of life.

The doctors involved engage all of their interpersonal skills, including empathy, delicacy, subtlety and sometimes assertiveness. Additionally they maintain an awareness of how the team is working. There will be teaching, cold facts and figures provided by their warm blooded patients providing the raw material, and there will be humour, which promotes good feeling between colleagues. When the mood turns jocular the dark cloud that hovered above them (following, say, a discussion with a patient about their cancer diagnosis), dissipates in an instant.

So many juxtapositions. Such inconsistency. Do we mean any of it?

Nimble

The ability to be emotionally nimble is crucial in medicine. That's because the typical day will involve numerous human situations, to which the doctor must adapt quickly. She must sense the timing of the situation and change their demeanour, their behaviour and the choice of words accordingly. It is not so much the need to be a comedian as to absorb, reflect and then take the lead according to the feelings that have been experienced. For, in critical or emotionally demanding situations, all will be looking to the doctor for their contributions and their judgement as to how to proceed.

So this leads onto the question, are doctors the supreme actors? And are they professionally insincere?

This article is, of course, written from the point of view of a health care practitioner. One could argue that this is the wrong way round, and that sincerity needs to be confirmed from the patient's point of view. Certainly, if a doctor fails in making an accurate assessment of an emotionally charged situation, and adopts the wrong tone, they will come across as insincere. He will fail. The successful doctor will always *appear* sincere, but the question is – does it really matter if they believe, and feel, what they are saying? After all, surely it is the end result, and the effect that the words have on a patient or family, that really matters, not the true quality of emotions within.

Two kinds of acting

Raj Persaud wrote a brief and entertaining article for BMJ Careers - 'Faking it'. He explained that…

Psychologists use the term "surface level emotional labour" to capture the fact that a large part of dealing with people at work is basically "faking it" or displaying emotions we don't actually feel, like feigning interest, sympathy, or understanding.

One of his references is an internet accessible paper by C´eleste Brotheridge and Alicia Grandey, 'Emotional Labor and Burnout: Comparing Two Perspectives of "People Work"' (2002). In this, the relationship between those types of acting (be they voluntary or involuntary) are related to the preservation of mental wellbeing in people who work in 'service industries'. Medicine features prominently in it. They explain acting in more detail:

(NB - for 'customers' read 'patients'!)

'Surface acting'

In surface acting, employees modify and control their emotional expressions. For example, employees may enhance or fake a smile when in a bad mood or interacting with a difficult customer. The inauthenticity of this surface-level process, showing expressions discrepant from feelings, is related to stress outcomes due to the internal tension and the physiological effort of suppressing true feelings.

...inauthentic [acting] over time may result in feeling detached not only from one's true feelings but also from other people's feelings, suggesting a relationship with the dimension of depersonalization. Feeling diminished personal accomplishment is also likely if the employee believes that the displays were not efficacious or were met with annoyance by customers. Thus, surface acting is expected to relate to all three dimensions of burnout.

'Deep acting'

Deep acting is the process of controlling internal thoughts and feelings to meet the mandated display rules. Emotions involve physiological arousal and cognitions, and deep acting works on modifying arousal or cognitions through a variety of techniques.

...doing "emotion work" was a way of decreasing a state of emotional dissonance and may also result in a feeling of accomplishment if the performance is effective. Thus, deep acting might not relate to emotional exhaustion because it minimizes the tension of dissonance.

Another accessible article, 'Reassessing the concept of emotional labour in student nurse education: role of link lecturers and mentors in a time of change' by Pam Smith and Benjamin Gray (Nursing Education Today, 2000), explores these specifically in relation to healthcare. They cite Arlie Hochschild, author of 'The Managed Heart' (University of California Press, Berkeley, 1983), which seems to form the basis of most studies into how we modulate our emotions in the workplace.

Defining emotional labour Hochschild suggests that emotional labour involves the induction or suppression of feeling in order to sustain an outward appearance that produces in others a sense of being cared for in a convivial safe place.

The idea of 'emotional labour' really does chime, for most healthcare professionals would agree that emotional exhaustion precedes physical exhaustion during a busy shift. Just the other day I said to a colleague, 'I've had three DNAR discussions on this ward round, I don't think I can manage another right now.' But, just as superficial acting is associated with 'burnout' (a paradoxical and counterintuitive findings one might think), deep acting appears to lead to true 'job satisfaction'. This also rings true. You really feel you've done some good when you dip into a person's difficult life, make a significant intervention, and then leave them. That is medicine. The satisfaction negates the exhaustion. It is 'dissonance' that wears you down.

Smith and Gray also note,

By brushing over the emotional labour of nurses as an essential skill that does not require development, because it is so 'basic', the techniques of nurses' emotional labour go unappreciated and are not developed as resources for the National Health Service (NHS) to draw upon.

This is a valuable comment. What seems like an 'obvious' element of compassionate healthcare is in fact a resource, one that is not infinite. A highly relevant point in the current climate of criticism.

An emotional continuum

We act. I think we can accept that as a given. It's part of our professional skill set. I am more interested in how this affects our ability to provide compassionate care. My suggestion, and I would love to know what others think about this, is that rather than flipping between a mere two levels of acting and involvement, we move steadily along a continuum, like whales plumbing the ocean depths, responding to our perception of how emotionally complex and ethically demanding each situation is. I can only speak for myself, but I think the 'emotional work' that I commit to is in direct proportion to those quotients. The expression of compassion is, in turn, directly related to that commitment, the words and actions being fuelled by a rarer and more precious fuel. The rewards however, are all the greater, as noted above. To put it simply, 'you get out what you put in'… but it is unrealistic to put in your all during every interaction.

A warning

So, what of our consultant, the one who said all the right things and then displayed a streak of cynicism to her junior a minute later? I think I understand her. She had become too nimble, too smooth, too adept at making the quick change in emotional depth. She, the consummate actor, found it too easy to flit between compassionate caregiver and amusing educator. However sincere her words to the patient's daughter, the rapid alteration in tone belied her.

Compassion in healthcare: the separation trap

The recent call for greater compassion in healthcare struck me as simplistic. Secretary of State Jeremy Hunt's demand for more personal warmth during medical and nursing interactions came across as a bemused and impatient plea – 'Why can't you just…be nice!' It was as though he could not understand why a typical doctor or nurse could be other than ever-smiling, spilling over with bonhomie, eager always to go the extra mile to make their patients' experience of hospital as pleasant as possible. Of course, this is not the case. Why?

Healthcare professionals (HCPs) are human. They have good days and bad days. Sometimes they don't like their jobs. And sadly, for patients, when HCPs are in a less than excellent mood the first thing to go is the soft, warm surface against which the sick are forced, by ill fortune, to rub. Underneath that surface lies the metallic functionality of a busy, hard pressed worker. Driven by a tight timetable, their day comprising a list of tasks that must be accomplished, the typical HCP will, at core, be efficient and task focused. And when the shift ends and the time comes to hand over to colleagues, it is the lack of completion, not the absence of human kindness that should have been woven into those tasks, that will be missed.

Or have I got this all the wrong way round? The paragraph above is clearly written by a task-focused HCP. I admit it – I have always preferred to finish a list of medical tasks than leave 20% hanging over to another day, or more likely, another colleague. Yes, even if that means the *quality* of those tasks is diluted, by which I mean the quality of the communication with which those tasks were framed.

So is this the choice that we present to our patients – efficiency *vs* compassion? It reminds me of the clichéd personality types depicted in medical fiction: who would you prefer, the brilliant and stitch perfect surgeon with few human skills, or her competent, but more empathetic colleague who did far less well in his exams? Is this really the choice?

No. Wrong again. The mistake that I have made here is in *separating* the task and the compassionate style with which it is performed. They belong to each other, and the one cannot be carried out successfully without the other. The overall task can certainly be broken down to component parts, but if the visible, human face of it is neglected it cannot be said to have been completed properly. Perhaps that 100% completion rate that doctors like me were trained aim for, achieving it by and large, was always a delusion; perhaps our training, by emphasising completion, led us to become satisfied with sub-optimal care, because that vital element, compassion, was undermined.

The tendency to separate process and compassion was brought home to me a little while ago. The ward round led my team to the bed of a middle aged man with a progressive neurological disorder that rendered his speech incredibly slow, while preserving his cognitive function. His thoughts were as clear as they had ever been. On this occasion I was up against the clock – there was a meeting in 15 minutes time and he was my penultimate patient. As soon as I approached the bed I remembered how difficult our interaction was likely to be, and in a business like way I summarised the results of recent investigations and the management plan. He nodded and managed a few words, slowly, indicating that he understood everything. I moved away from the bed but paused as I heard him form the first syllable of another word. Of course I had no choice but to wait for him to complete the sentence. And that sentence was just part of a series of sentences which he had undoubtedly been considering all morning.

He wished to enlarge our discussion to explore options for future care in the community. For half a minute I attempted to finish his sentences for him, the phrases and idioms being instantly recognisable. Aware of how rude and patronizing this must seem I stopped, allowing him to complete each sentence while I swiftly composed my answer and, in the many spare seconds, controlled my growing agitation about the meeting to which I was committed. He continued.

I looked down at my feet. My body language indicated haste and impatience. I was still two steps away from the bed and standing at such an angle that it was clear I had been arrested mid-stride. Perhaps he was used to this, for he continued in a calm and measured way. I saw myself and saw how poorly I must be coming across. The interaction that had started on my terms now continued on his. I relaxed, approached the bed and closed my mind to other matters. The subject of the conversation was not particularly delicate or ethically complex. There was no great emotional unburdening, no breaking of bad news. He just needed to discuss something with his consultant. From my point of view the business of his medical management had been dealt with in a moment, but from his point of view there was more to do.

The clock ticked on, he imparted the information, told me his opinion…I responded, we had a conversation. And as I walked away, 10 minutes late for my meeting, I reflected that although I had been obliged to change my attitude and soften my style, if only for a short time, it had required quite a lot of effort. It had required me to mentally disengage from the business of the day and carve out a piece of time. I congratulated myself for the compassion I had shown, but then ridiculed myself for such shallow thinking. Although I felt that I had been especially 'kind', in fact I had done nothing more than be polite and had show respect to another person for quarter of an hour. And if I had walked away, having decided to ignore the effortful, muted syllable that was just the beginning of a long string of sentences, I would have denied him the chance to talk in depth with the person in charge of his care. So what seemed like a marvellous example of compassion to me was no more than a basic aspect of medical care to him.

This all seems well and good. If you begin an interaction with a patient you must commit to conducting it with compassion. But there is a sting in the tail. I was 25 minutes late to the meeting, one in which important matters were due to be discussed, where decisions were due to be taken that would in the end contribute to improved care for many other patients. So, bearing that in mind, should I have hurried off, with the justification that the needs of the many outweigh the needs of the few, or the one? Should the hard pressed ward nurse hurry from one patient to the next with barely a word, in order to serve the many rather than the few, within the allotted time?

The answer to this is a little easier to find when it is approached from the patient's point of view. My patient, the 'painfully' slow talker who was desperate to explore important, if non-urgent personal matters, had no care for my timetable, my 'commitments', nor for the welfare of other patients, either present or future. He was focused on *his* situation and *his* relationship with *his* consultant. And that is the essence of the matter. Patients remember what happened to *them*, and are not cognizant of their small role in the complex, churning, leviathan structure of the hospital. Why should they be? They want medical efficiency and accuracy, but care greatly for the feel of things. Memories are coloured not by results or shortened stays in hospital, but by the tenor and the warmth of interactions with medical staff.

The visit: an interrogation of caring

Night.

Patient: "A few weeks ago you promised to do something for me, when I saw you in clinic. Do you remember?"

Doctor: "I recognise your face. I think I remember…"

"Barely! You promised to check my blood results. You were worried that my kidneys were failing, and you said I might have to come into hospital."

"Yes, yes…what happened?"

"You didn't ring, I presume you didn't check. I called an ambulance on the third day because I was feeling so bad. They took me straight in. You should have seen the look on the young doctor's face, she was horrified. She said she had never seen so much acid in someone's blood stream…"

"Oh."

"You were right. I had bad renal failure."

"I'm sorry."

"We'll get to that."

"What happened."

"I was rushed into intensive care to go on a kidney machine…but it was too late."

"What do you mean?"

"I heard the consultant say to one of the other doctors that I was too far gone. Too late."

"I don't…"

"I died. Hasn't it sunk in yet? I died! You're asleep, and I've come to interrogate you. Or perhaps you're interrogating yourself, driven by guilt. It doesn't matter really. I get to ask my questions either way. One. Why didn't you do what you promised?"

"I remember you now. I was worried, but I had no way of telling it was that advanced…"

"The bloods would have told you, if you'd looked them up next day. Want to hear my theory?"

"Go on."

"It was because you didn't really care…"

"Of course I cared. I was worried about you."

"Not enough. You think you cared about me because I was sitting in front of you, my problem was filling your vision…but as soon as I left you began to worry about other people with more immediate problems. If you cared about me, it was for a few moments."

"I remember our conversation. I asked about you, about your family, I didn't treat you like a number or a 'case'."

"You were nice to me, yes. You came across very caring. That's why I went home satisfied, feeling safe and looked after. But you know what, I would rather you had actually cared enough to protect me after I left the room. I wish that caring had been strong enough to keep my problems near the front of your mind next day…so you wouldn't forget. That way, I might be alive now."

"You're mixing up the types of care…the care we feel for people, emotions, and the care we provide."

"Oh, you've hit it. Right on the head. That's my whole point. The care you and your colleagues provide is physical, keeping us clean, fed, warm, dry…giving us medicine. That's the basics. But I think the care you give would be better if you actually cared about us. If you cared about me, personally, perhaps you would have checked my results. You would have come to work and I would have been on your mind. My fate, my wellbeing, would have been bugging you. That's the weakness you see, in giving others power over you. If they don't care, they won't think about you when you are out of sight."

"Is it reasonable, to expect a doctor to truly care about all the people he or she sees?"

"But aren't you trained to care? Aren't you supposed to communicate warmth, empathy, a caring attitude? That's what you did with me, misleading me. You made me feel as though I was at the centre of your thoughts, and I was naïve enough to believe it. Of course you weren't going to rush in to check my results next day, you weren't going to put aside your other commitments, delay seeing the visibly ill patients on your ward…"

"So you think the caring I showed you was what? Fake?"

"Just shallow."

"Insincere perhaps. Come on, this can't get any worse."

"A form of narcissism. That's what I think."

"What?! What do you mean by that?"

"I think that the attitude or behaviour that you display at work is professionalised. It is doing what is required of you, what's expected, and what keeps us happy. You listen to yourself, the tone seems right, the words appropriate, yes…I'm doing this right you say to yourself. Perhaps you even believe yourself. You reassure yourself that you are a nice person. Sensitive. And then....you go home and forget us."

"That's not true."

"Really. You think about us outside the hospital? I do not believe that. Tell me, honestly, when was the last time you went home and dwelt on a patient, and worried not about the medical decision, but about the person?"

"It happens! I'm telling you it happens."

"Yes, I believe you. I believe you because of the way you said it just then. You meant it, you tapped into an emotional scar. Someone you had looked after for a long time, someone with a particularly tragic story? Someone young? Someone who reminded you of a loved one? Not a typical patient though. Bur that's not good enough, to reserve your caring for the odd one."

"Many patients have got under my skin."

"Like parasites you mean! You can't live with hundreds, thousands, living under your skin, can you? But if they have to get under your skin for you to care about them, and not forget to do the little things that you promised them, how can you provide the personalised, tailored care that you pretend to offer when they sit just a foot away from you?"

"I'm not having this. I do care. I feel sad whenever a patient of mine suffers."

"No. No, no, no. Sadness does not derive from caring."

"It does. If I didn't care why would I react with a kind of grief – short-lived I admit, but real."

"I think the feeling that you experience is complex. You worry that they have suffered because you've messed up, or missed something. Just as you felt when I visited you tonight. That was your first thought…Shit! What did I do wrong. Wasn't it? You might worry that the suffering indicates a deterioration, the possibility of death. That will make you sad, as it would any normal human being. But I don't think that sadness will stay with you beyond the confines of the hospital. That's not how you react to someone you care about. Is it?"

"Perhaps it's not so rare as you think. You know less about doctors than you think."

"I'm sure there may be the odd one the doctor has grown to like, even to bond with. But I think that's a rare thing indeed. Let's approach this another way, if you had time. Imagine we haven't started this conversation, in fact imagine I met you on the street, imagine I was conducting a sociological survey. And I said, could you care about. What would you have said? Now be honest."

"I guess my thoughts would have immediately focused on my family."

"And if pressed?"

"Then I would've begun to think about a few particular friends."

"Yes, that's normal. Those are the ones you care about. Then still you insist that you care about your patients? Stop pretending. You don't, not really. You have trained yourself to say that you do, because to say otherwise would seem callous. But be honest, with me of all people. I'm sorry, I don't mean to distress you. But I want to get the truth."

"Perhaps we need to consider different types of caring."

"Yes, that's where I was coming from all the time. Professional caring. Shallow caring. If it's the best you can do, admit it. The thing is doctor, I really don't care if you care. I only care about you doing your job, yes in caring way, and properly, but I'm not bothered if my problems play on your mind. The motivation behind your actions doesn't bother me. Perhaps you'll be nice to me, and I'll have a good experience, if you care about me, but, understanding the depth of feeling behind your professionalism doesn't make a huge difference. Feel what I'm feeling, empathise, in order to treat me better, yes, but use it as a tool. Dip into my emotional world, don't inhabit it. But please…if you make a promise, do it."

"I'm sorry, for what I didn't do."

"Forget it. Perhaps it never happened.

Part 3: At the coalface

Hazard in context: the psychology of medical continuity

Continuity of care in hospital is a hot topic. It is well recognised that reductions in the hours worked by junior doctors have resulted in a fracturing of the traditional team structure and more frequent handovers between staff as they come off shorter shifts. The Royal College of Physicians published a survey on the subject in February 2012, their press release saying,

'...over a quarter (28%) of consultant physicians surveyed rate their hospital's ability to deliver continuity of care as poor or very poor. In addition, over a quarter (27%) believe that their hospital is poor or very poor at delivering stable medical teams for patient care and education.'

Although improved safety on the wards was a driver for change, a document published by the Royal College of Surgeons, '*Do reduced doctors' working hours create better safety for patients? – assessing the evidence*', challenged the assumption that working to the European Working Time Directive (48 rather than 56) led to greater alertness and fewer mistakes. The author Matthew Worral wrote,

'There is a much greater evidence base to suggest the full-shift system being brought in increases patient harm through greater handovers and stratification of hospital staff. The potential for important information to be missed and inability to access senior expertise at key times are a greater problem for patients.'

Accompanying the move from long on-call periods to shifts has been a reconfiguration of the way patients are assigned to teams. In a soon to be published book 'The Changing Role of Doctors' (Radcliffe Health, May 2013), the main strength of the 'old way' is neatly described;

'This firm structure, with the associated working pattern, meant there was a high level of understanding of one another's strengths, weaknesses, training needs and personality. When this medical team was working at its best, all members of staff felt supported and there was a genuine sense of camaraderie and team spirit.'

and,

'Continuity of patient care was of a very high level. Most patients were clerked in by a member of a firm (usually the most junior doctor) and then remained under the same team of doctors for the duration of the stay, regardless of where the available beds were.'

This contrasts with the new 'ward based' model, where,

'...the junior doctor and consultant who first admit a patient will usually pass over the responsibility of care for the patient to another team as soon as the patient moves to an inpatient ward.'

The ward based model has significant strengths, not the least of which is that patients are directed to teams with expertise in their particular disease, rather than remaining with the 'random' team who happened to be on-call on the day they were admitted. Another strength is that work intensity remains constant, rather than fluctuating with the ebb and flow of admissions either side of an on-call day. A major downside is that whenever the patient moves within the hospital (into a side room because of infective diarrhoea, for example), her or she becomes the responsibility of *another* team. That team will have to review all that has gone before, check the results, get up to speed, and carry on delivering appropriate care seamlessly. The process of developing a full understanding of the patient's needs and goals must be repeated. Rapport must be rebuilt. Subtleties may be lost. Errors can be made.

What is at the heart of these errors? System failures, 'dropped batons', poor communication...all are likely contributors. Professor Roy Pounder, contemplating the effects of reduced working hours, <u>highlighted these factors in advance of the EWTD</u> <u>changes:</u>

"Seeing a patient once or twice before handing over to the next doctor, who then does the same after a short period, means it is difficult to detect a subtle deterioration in a patient's condition."

But I wonder if there is a deeper issue, related to the way doctors understand their patients. The psychology of discontinuity. This needs to be addressed from the point of view of both patients and doctors.

Patient experience: anchorage

A 2002 BMJ paper, '<u>Continuity of hospital care: beyond the</u> <u>question of personal contact</u>' offered some good insights into patient experience, using the following quotes;

"They keep asking the same questions..."

"My file was not present and new doctors were not informed of my situation"

"You always get different orders from new doctors"

"Too many doctors! A second opinion is OK, but the sixth and seventh are quite frustrating..."

These are the more obvious symptoms of discontinuity, but they do not describe fully the sense of vulnerability and frustration that I have sometimes detected. When I see a patient in the emergency department or acute admissions ward, a common question is,

"Are you going to be my doctor now?"

or,

"Will you be coming back to see me again? Will I see you tomorrow?"

I interpret such questions as an appeal for permanence or anchorage in the huge, complex system into which they have been delivered. Patients, it seems to me, are desperate to make a connection that can be relied on. If I know that the patient will come to my ward, I can answer 'Yes, I'll be along to see you tomorrow...' and there may be a visible relaxation in their anxious expression. But if not, I have no choice but to explain, 'No, it won't be me who sees you from now on...but one of the other teams, lung specialists...' Sometimes, if I have spent a good deal of time speaking with them, digging down in important medical or social details, I will add, 'But we will make sure they know all about you...about everything we have discussed...' If it is a crucial fact I will make a point of telling the new team, but more often than not such hand-over of information will occur on paper, in the notes. This requires a clear handwritten entry, a transparent narrative. It is not uncommon for me to see what has been written by the junior doctor accompanying me only to realise that they have not interpreted the patient's words in the same way I have.

The emphasis is not quite right. So I re-write it, and leave the ward hoping and expecting that whoever receives that patient will see my note and make sense of it. This is an attempt to maintain the chain of continuity.

I wonder if the psychological distress that derives from uncertainty, not knowing if someone in the machine 'owns' you, if someone is personally invested in your wellbeing, may be sufficient to undo the benefit of technically correct, well timed medical interventions.

Fast track empathy

How do lack of continuity and the diminished feeling of ownership that follows, influence doctors in a way that jeopardises safety? It may hinge on empathy.

Serious illness requires the application of powerful medical interventions. These bring with them the potential for hazard. Recent debate about 'zero harm' culture has crystallised the notion that medicine and its tools can do as much harm as good. To avoid harm staff must be vigilant; they need to keep an eye on the details, spot irregularities, check the blood tests, double check the drug charts, maintain the 'housekeeping' (as it is sometimes called), and anticipate complications. These duties should be automatic, but they are done better if the doctor knows the full story. If they have gained a full appreciation of the patient and their background they will understand better the true impact of those potential harms.

Risks and harms can appear abstract, but when they are imagined in the context of the whole person they become tangible, transforming from theoretical 'adverse events' to personal tragedies. A better understanding of those risks may motivate doctors to work harder in ensuring that each job is done properly. Otherwise they will not be letting down, '…the lady in bed 25, acute kidney injury…', but 'Mrs Jones…she was hoping to get out in time to attend her grand-daughter's wedding this weekend…' Continuity encourages personalisation, personalisation permits the exercise of empathy, and empathy gives our actions relevance.

The challenge for doctors working to shift patterns and caring for patients who arrive to their ward areas on a daily basis, is to learn the practise of empathy in compressed timeframes. This requires active listening, generous emotional investment…energy. But to ensure that connections between patients and doctors are made within the restrictions of the modern hospital environment this has to happen. Otherwise patients will flow through wards without knowing if anyone really 'owned' them, or who that person was. And doctors will float from patient to patient without understanding quite how much trust was being put in them.

When paternalism = bravery: a 'slow code' dilemma

What are doctors supposed to do if a patient's relatives fail to agree with a Do Not Resuscitate order, even when the doctor knows that such resuscitation would be completely futile? One solution to this, described in literature coming out of the United States, is the 'slow code'. This is when a deliberately ineffectual resuscitation attempt is made to satisfy relatives, but also to ensure that on no account will a patient's heart be restarted. 'Code' is the American term for a crash call. A 2011 paper in the American Journal of Bioethics (£) defended this practice, albeit in the arena of neonatology where the positive psychological effect on parents who need to know that 'everything was done' may be more important.

"A leading textbook calls slow codes 'dishonest, crass dissimulation, and unethical.' A medical sociologist describes them as 'deplorable, dishonest and inconsistent with established ethical principles.' Nevertheless, we believe that slow codes may be appropriate and ethically defensible in situations in which cardiopulmonary resuscitation (CPR) is likely to be ineffective, the family decision makers understand and accept that death is inevitable, and those family members cannot bring themselves to consent or even assent to a do-not-resuscitate (DNR) order."

Another paper, based on interviews with critical care practitioners ("Slow" Code: Perspectives of a Physician and Critical Care Nurse, Critical Care Nursing Quarterly 1999) [free access] included this powerful passage:

"I remember a specific case involving a 30-year-old patient with a particularly virulent strain of pneumonia. Blood was sent to NIH to rule out hanta virus. It was a case that was frightening but also very enlightening and interesting. She developed full-blown ARDS so severe that only bilateral lung transplants would have saved her.

"Routine turning caused her to desaturate because she was that unstable. I can understand that, because she was 30 years old, the family wanted everything done. No matter what we said to them, they didn't hear that there were no alternatives. Of course, this was an extreme case, one in which I can understand the family's wishes.

"If I didn't have the medical knowledge about ARDS and someone told me that my 30-year-old sister was going to die, I would have wanted everything done. The family thought we could do lung transplants right there in the room. They had to be very gently wooed into the idea of a DNR status. She coded before a DNR status could be obtained. In this case, the family was very

much opposed to a DNR status and a "slow" code was performed to satisfy their needs."

In acute general medicine similar but less dramatic dilemmas are encountered on a daily basis. Although it is rare for disagreements between relatives and doctors to arise, it is common for there to be a delay of several days while families engage in conversations about the benefits, and burdens, of resuscitation. During that hiatus, anything could happen. Many patients therefore remain For Resuscitation, by default, while doctors attempt to achieve consensus.

Consider this scenario. A 91 year old lady is admitted to hospital with symptoms of urinary tract infection and significant kidney dysfunction. She is confused, temporarily, by the sepsis. She has been living alone but depending on the help of relatives and neighbours, nothing major. The consultant agrees with the junior doctor's initial diagnosis and confirms that the antibiotic and fluid prescriptions are correct. There is no sign of cardiac instability, but he decides to take the relatives (a son and a daughter, in their late 50's or 60's) to one side. He begins to explore the subject of unexpected complications, and the possibility of sudden cardiac arrest.

'I'd like to discuss with you on the issue of resuscitation. Your mother doesn't appear to be in any danger, but we must consider that during any illness there is a risk of sudden deterioration. We should anticipate what we should do, and what she would want us to do, if heart were to stop.'

'She's very strong. She was ill four years with pneumonia but she pulled through, she's a fighter.'

'I can see she is, but if the worst were to happen, and the heart were to stop, then however strong she seems now it would be very difficult for her to recover.'

'So what are you saying?'

'My feeling is that the chances of her coming round, of surviving, even if we did cardiac compressions and gave electric shocks with the defibrillator, the chances would be very small. I think she would have a lot of damage to the heart and possibly the brain, and would be unlikely to leave hospital.'

'We haven't really thought about this before. No one has ever said this before.'

'I'm not asking you to decide, certainly not. It's just important that you understand why we make these decisions, and important that we know how your mother would feel.'

'What would your advice be?'

'I definitely would not advise that she has resuscitation. I would be very uncomfortable letting that happen given her physical frailty.'

The doctor recognises a steely look in the two relative's eyes. He senses that his introduction of the subject of dying has caused a reaction. They exchange glances, and the son replies,

'Well we really do have to go away and talk about that. I mean, as I say, she would want everything possible done to get her through this. She really is a fighter. She had a cancer operation five years ago, and they said she couldn't have that...but she did.'

'OK. I don't think we have to reach a final decision at this precise time. Perhaps it's good that we've talked about this now...you can think about it with the family overnight. But my opinion would be that resuscitation would not be right for her. Perhaps tomorrow or the next day we can talk again...I really would like there to be something in her notes so that any other medical teams called to see her know what to do if...she goes downhill.'

'Fine. But we need to talk about this as a family.'

The junior doctor, who was present throughout, asks,

'But isn't it a medical decision?'

'Yes it is. You're quite right. But do *you* want to tell them that, at the moment? They are shocked by the idea that their mother might die. I think it's a step too far tonight to write a Do Not Resuscitate form until they have expressed their agreement.'

'But if she does arrest you've said she won't survive. As it stands she'll be resuscitated if she arrests.'

'My assessment is that the risk is low. If she was showing signs of instability I would probably have to force the issue tonight, and perhaps write out a DNAR form without their agreement. But it's going to take a lot of talking to lead them to understand the reasons why we don't want to resuscitate.'

So the form goes unwritten. The consultant leaves in the hope that nothing untoward will happen. Has he done the right thing?

Here are some potential futures.

- Outcome [1] -

The patient has cardiac arrest at 2 o'clock in the morning. The crash team is called and begins to work on her. While the anaesthetist prepares to intubate another doctor performs cardiac compressions, and the nurse attaches defibrillator pads to her chest. The medical registrar, standing at the end of the bed, reads through the notes. There is very little to read, only the admission clerking and the post take ward round entry. There are no major co-morbidities, but the patient's advanced age and her evident physical frailty are inescapable. The second bolus of adrenaline is just about to be given when the registrar puts her hand up and says, 'I don't think this is right. The consultant was hoping to make her Not For Resus but the patient but the family didn't agree. He wrote that it's to be reviewed tomorrow. Clearly he thought she shouldn't be For. There's no way she's going to survive this. We should probably stop. Does everybody agree?'

The anaesthetist nods, the nurse running the ward nods. There is agreement… and the attempt is stopped.

What harm was done here?

The patient died and was not aware of anything. There was a genuine attempt to revive her, but, as soon as the registrar became aware of the circumstances she stopped it. Not a slow code, but a short code; almost an accidental code.

So, although the patient remained For Resuscitation, according to the paperwork, she was Not For Resuscitation, in spirit. The intention of the consultant who could not bring himself to actually fill out the form was in fact carried through by the crash team, although the patient still suffered (unconsciously) the indignity of three minutes of full-on advanced cardiac life support.

This strikes me as duplicitous. The decision not to resuscitate, very likely correct, had been made but had not been enacted or formalised for fear of resistance from the family. It is reasonable in this case that the form was not filled out because the consultant thought there was only a low risk of the patient dying over the next 24 hours, but...but, patients in their 90s do sadly die without warning. So the sensible precaution not to resuscitate was not in place. The reason? The consultant did not want to find himself at odds with the family, or the subject of a complaint. Because another scenario is as follows...

- Outcome [2] -

As the consultant departed from the ward round he had second thoughts. His junior's question had got to him. So he went back, explained his reasons in the notes and completed the Do Not Resuscitate form. He felt that this was the right thing to for the patient. The patient arrested at 2 o'clock in the morning. The nurses had been informed of the DNAR decision and the crash team were not called. The patient died quite suddenly but quite peacefully. The family were called, after death, given its unexpected nature. They arrived, asked about the circumstances, and learned that no attempt had been made to revive her. They were upset; voices were raised. Three weeks later and formal complaint was made.

The consultant had unilaterally made the patient Not For Resuscitation, in opposition to the families interpretation of their mother's desires, desires that she might have able to articulate had she had not been temporarily confused by the infection.

Without going over the top here, I am tempted to portray the consultant's actions in Outcome [2] as brave. In order to protect his patient from the risk of a futile resuscitation attempt he signed the form, did the 'right thing' (according to his analysis of the situation), but took a risk. He knew that there was a chance of generating a complaint, of being accused of paternalism, arrogance and playing God.

What would you do?

Notes:

i) GMC guidelines for DNAR decisions in patients who lack capacity to be involved in the decision emphasise the desirability of involving the healthcare team and those close to the patient, in order to understand as much as possible about the patient, and their known attitudes. However, as regards family agreement,

"In particular, you should be clear about the role that others are being asked to take in the decision-making process. If they do not have legal authority to make the decision, you should be clear that their role is to advise you and the healthcare team about the patient. You must not give them the impression that it is their

responsibility to decide whether CPR will be of overall benefit to the patient."

ii) Why not try to resuscitate a 91 year old lady? The literature suggests that very few patients in this age range survive to discharge. Although age in isolation is never used to decide on treatment, the fact remains that overall fragility and organ function is likely to be impaired at this stage of life. For specific citations on this subject see a previous blog, 'A form of words: honesty, kindness, coercion and early resuscitation discussions.'

iii) Most physicians I know would *not* fill out the DNAR form in this scenario.

What we talk about when we talk about death: a case

An elderly man, the precise age is immaterial, is admitted from home having had a fall. It is quickly determined that he has a chest infection, and antibiotics are started. We are optimistic that he will recover. On the second day he appears confused, and the amount of oxygen he requires goes up. Sometimes people get worse before they get better, and the antibiotics have barely got into his system...we carry on. We know now that despite his jovial character and bluff attitude, he was not in such good shape at home. He managed on his own, but the neighbours did all the shopping and he was rarely seen out of the house. He smoked two packs of cigarettes a day, always had done, as evidenced by his yellow hair, leathery skin and walnut coloured fingertips. His lungs are overlarge, expanded, most of the air-sacs within broken down and useless.

On the third day we begin to worry. A blood test that is used to track the progress of an infection (CRP, not infallible) has gone up, from 60 to 150. We ring the microbiologist for advice, essentially for permission to use a stronger antibiotic. These are commonly effective, but bring with them the risk of Clostridium *difficile*, a potentially lethal diarrhoea bug. We prescribe it.

We haven't seen any relatives, but I ask my team to make sure that his next-of-kin, whoever it is, knows that things are not going so well. On the fourth day he looks a little better, on the fifth worse. He isn't eating well, and we worry that poor nutrition will hinder his recovery. I ask a nurse to insert a feeding tube, but he pulls it out half an hour later. Another is inserted, carefully taped down, but he wriggles a finger underneath and yanks it out. Third time lucky…we secure the tube with a 'bridle', a small clip that attaches the tube to a piece of string that runs into one nostril and out of the other. It is now impossible for him to pull out the tube without traumatising his own nasal septum. The bridle is a standard technique, and not as unkind as it sounds. Thankfully, he stops pulling the tube and starts to receive proper sustenance.

On the sixth day we are told that his oxygen levels have fallen again. Another x-ray shows that the white shadow, the patch of pneumonia, has enlarged to occupy half the left lung. The new antibiotic has not worked. We make a decision – on the 'ceiling of care'. We must decide, for the benefit of all who might be called to see him 'out of hours', how far things should go.

We have a high dependency ward, where he can be more closely monitored and receive assisted ventilation with a portable machine. The next step, should that fail, would be intensive care. That is a big step. It is run by another group of doctors the 'intensivists', who must agree that the patient is a 'good candidate', ie. has a reasonable chance of surviving. The treatments they can provide are often miraculous, but they are also invasive. In cases of severe pneumonia the only real option is to sedate the patient, insert a tube into the trachea, or windpipe, and do all the breathing for them. But to recover from this period of complete physical dependence one needs a reserve of bodily strength. Patients weaken on ICU and to admit someone when you know that the chance of recovery is slight is hard to justify. Not only do they need to be strong enough to survive the actual infection, they must have enough lung function left to allow the ventilator to be detached before it causes its own complications. Then they must be able to get back on their legs and back home to live a tolerable life. This is no easy judgement, and must be done without bringing your own set of values to their projected quality of life. It is safer to just concentrate on the physical recovery and whether they will survive or not.

We make a decision that going on a mechanical ventilator is a step too far. He is transferred to the high dependency ward and a tight mask is placed around the nose and mouth so that the portable ventilator can push oxygen enriched air into his lungs under pressure. We review all of the blood results and cultures and see if the culpable bacteria can be identified, but there are no clues. There are stronger antibiotics out there but we keep our faith with the second line choice.

Next day he is barely conscious. For some reason the chest infection has advanced through the lung despite everything we have done. I begin to wonder whether the 'burden' of treatment is justified if the truth is that he cannot survive this illness. And this is where we begin to discuss end of life management. If it is clear that he cannot survive based on the fragility of his lungs and the rapidity of the advancing infection perhaps it would be kinder to stop pretending that we can reverse things and start to think about his comfort.

We meet with his son has now come down from the north of the country. It is clear that the relationship is not a straightforward one. He has not seen his father for 18 months, and the interaction is not a particularly loving one, I can tell. Not all families function according to the ideal. The son is clearly uncomfortable during the discussion, as though we are asking him what to do. That is not the intention. We need him to understand the reasons for our decisions to make sure that he does not strongly object, and to allow him to tell us what his father might have wanted. He agrees with our plan.

So at the end of the 8th day we surrender, on the patient's behalf, to the illness that was once called 'old man's friend'. A nurse detaches the mask and rests his head back against the pillow. We look at the drug chart and cross off the antibiotics that were intended to save him. He has a small tube one of his wrist arteries and I instruct the nurse to remove it. We request that he has no more blood tests and that the only injections he receives are those that make him more comfortable. I write up small doses of morphine and midazolam, a painkiller and sedative, to be used if he appears to be distressed. If his cannula comes out he will not have another one inserted, even if this means he does not get any extra fluids. His veins have become thready and bruised, it would take the junior doctor four or five attempts to get one in. The drugs that he may need can be injected under the skin.

We start the Liverpool Care Pathway. In this way any doctor or nurse asked to see him overnight will not have to guess at our intentions and conclusions, but will know that active or 'heroic' treatment is not appropriate. He is, of course, made DNAR...for after all, we have accepted that his heart will soon stop and any attempt to restart it would be indefensible. But even at this point I ask myself – are missing a chance to save him? He was clearly a tough chap. A week and half ago he was living alone, happy, doing the things that amused him. He hardly ever saw a doctor, as shown by the slim medical folder that has been retrieved from records. The cigarettes had never really bothered him. Perhaps if we continued to treat, or if we reached for the even stronger antibiotic, we might yet reverse the infection. Nothing is certain. Would the patient want us to continue with this aggressive policy in the face of almost certain failure? Would he want his sore nose and chin to be continually rubbed by the tight mask, to have blood tests twice a day, the feeding tube in his nostril, if the chance of success is only 5%...or less? I don't know. His son doesn't know. We make the decision because we have seen this situation hundreds, thousands of times.

Perhaps, by stopping the antibiotic, we will let the infection progress more rapidly still. Perhaps, by stopping the fluids, his blood pressure will go down and his heart stop a little earlier. Perhaps the tiny dose of morphine that he receives overnight will slow his breathing even more, bringing forward the final collapse. It is possible that he may survive another four days if we continue aggressive therapy, but only one day on the LCP. But those extra days will be full of discomfort, and that suffering will achieve nothing. Those three days will represent the prolongation of death, not life.

[This case is fictional]

Medicus Mendax: false final words

I have been in this position a few times now. To protect confidentiality, the following account is inspired by a number of experiences and does not describe a specific patient.

A young patient, well known to me, was admitted to the hospital once again. She had become severely jaundiced and the cause, as usual, was heavy drinking. Just a month ago she had spent three weeks in hospital being fed via a nasal tube and receiving steroid tablets to calm down the dangerous inflammation in her liver. This time she was even more unwell. Her arms and legs were thin, her abdomen was swollen and she was confused. But, as before, after a few days her strength began to return and the jaundice improved. Her family came in. They tried to convince her to stay at home with them in order watch over her, but she preferred to live in a shared house, with her friends, friends who supplied her with alcohol.

As I left one night I saw her sister walk onto the ward. 'Pretty stable.' I told her. We knew that she was unlikely to survive more than six months given the gradual decline in liver function, but the time that she spent outside hospital was satisfactory to her, and not without pleasure, or freedom. We had made every effort to help her recover from alcoholism, but to no avail.

As I drove in one morning I received a phone call to say that she had vomited two pints of blood on the ward. I parked the car and rushed in, knowing that she would need to be admitted to the intensive care unit for resuscitation and an emergency endoscopy. She lay on her side, a puddle of congealing blood extending from her head to her chest on the bed sheet. The floor was sticky with it. She was groaning, but still conscious, fully aware of what was going on. The curtains had been pulled around all the other patients' beds so that they did not have to witness this terrible scene.

Within fifteen minutes she had been transferred to the intensive care unit and preparations were made to sedate and intubate her. This would allow me to perform an endoscopy without her struggling and moving around. I stood over her and she looked up. I explained what we were planning to do. She said, 'Doctor, just tell me I'm going to wake up from this.' I hesitated and said, 'Yes, we should be able to stop the bleeding and stabilise you, you should be awake in a couple of days.' An oxygen mask was put over her face and the first sedative was administered.

I had lied to her. I knew her liver was probably not strong enough to sustain her through this massive haemorrhage. Privately I gave her a 10 to 20% chance, at most, of pulling through. A large enough chance to justify aggressive treatment, especially for such a young patient, but a long shot. As the anaesthetist began to insert the endotracheal tube a dark fountain rose up from her mouth and poured onto the already sodden pillow. Twin rivulets of blood fell from her nostrils. Her hair was matted with it.

When I passed the endoscope into her oesophagus all I could see was red. I then inserted a balloon into the stomach to squeeze the engorged vessels from below, but her blood had become too thin and she continued to bleed. I tensed the balloon as much as possible, but over the next two hours she lost more blood and her heart began to fail. The family arrived and I spoke with them. Death was now certain. She died half an hour later. It was no surprise – not to me, not to the nurses, not to the other consultants who looked after her in the past. But I could not forget that one of her last human interactions was with me, when I gave her reassurance that she would survive. I wonder if, as the sedatives kicked in, and the sound and the meaning of my words drifted across her darkening mind, they offered any comfort at all.

Hazard in context: the psychology of medical continuity

Continuity of care in hospital is a hot topic. It is well recognised that reductions in the hours worked by junior doctors have resulted in a fracturing of the traditional team structure and more frequent handovers between staff as they come off shorter shifts. The Royal College of Physicians published a survey on the subject in February 2012, their press release saying,

'...over a quarter (28%) of consultant physicians surveyed rate their hospital's ability to deliver continuity of care as poor or very poor. In addition, over a quarter (27%) believe that their hospital is poor or very poor at delivering stable medical teams for patient care and education.'

Although improved safety on the wards was a driver for change, a document published by the Royal College of Surgeons, 'Do reduced doctors' working hours create better safety for patients? – assessing the evidence', challenged the assumption that working to the European Working Time Directive (48 rather than 56) led to greater alertness and fewer mistakes. The author Matthew Worral wrote,

'There is a much greater evidence base to suggest the full-shift system being brought in increases patient harm through greater handovers and stratification of hospital staff. The potential for important information to be missed and inability to access senior expertise at key times are a greater problem for patients.'

Accompanying the move from long on-call periods to shifts has been a reconfiguration of the way patients are assigned to teams. In a soon to be published book <u>'The Changing Role of Doctors'</u> <u>(Radcliffe Health, May 2013)</u>, the main strength of the 'old way' is neatly described;

'This firm structure, with the associated working pattern, meant there was a high level of understanding of one another's strengths, weaknesses, training needs and personality. When this medical team was working at its best, all members of staff felt supported and there was a genuine sense of camaraderie and team spirit.'

and,

'Continuity of patient care was of a very high level. Most patients were clerked in by a member of a firm (usually the most junior doctor) and then remained under the same team of doctors for the duration of the stay, regardless of where the available beds were.'

This contrasts with the new 'ward based' model, where,

'...the junior doctor and consultant who first admit a patient will usually pass over the responsibility of care for the patient to another team as soon as the patient moves to an inpatient ward.'

The ward based model has significant strengths, not the least of which is that patients are directed to teams with expertise in their particular disease, rather than remaining with the 'random' team who happened to be on-call on the day they were admitted. Another strength is that work intensity remains constant, rather than fluctuating with the ebb and flow of admissions either side of an on-call day. A major downside is that whenever the patient moves within the hospital (into a side room because of infective diarrhoea, for example), her or she becomes the responsibility of another team. That team will have to review all that has gone before, check the results, get up to speed, and carry on delivering appropriate care seamlessly. The process of developing a full understanding of the patient's needs and goals must be repeated. Rapport must be rebuilt. Subtleties may be lost. Errors can be made.

What is at the heart of these errors? System failures, 'dropped batons', poor communication...all are likely contributors. Professor Roy Pounder, contemplating the effects of reduced working hours, highlighted these factors in advance of the EWTD changes:

"Seeing a patient once or twice before handing over to the next doctor, who then does the same after a short period, means it is difficult to detect a subtle deterioration in a patient's condition."

But I wonder if there is a deeper issue, related to the way doctors understand their patients. The psychology of discontinuity. This needs to be addressed from the point of view of both patients and doctors.

Patient experience: anchorage

A 2002 BMJ paper, 'Continuity of hospital care: beyond the question of personal contact' offered some good insights into patient experience, using the following quotes;

"They keep asking the same questions…"

"My file was not present and new doctors were not informed of my situation"

"You always get different orders from new doctors"

"Too many doctors! A second opinion is OK, but the sixth and seventh are quite frustrating…"

These are the more obvious symptoms of discontinuity, but they do not describe fully the sense of vulnerability and frustration that I have sometimes detected. When I see a patient in the emergency department or acute admissions ward, a common question is,

"Are you going to be my doctor now?"

or,

"Will you be coming back to see me again? Will I see you tomorrow?"

I interpret such questions as an appeal for permanence or anchorage in the huge, complex system into which they have been delivered. Patients, it seems to me, are desperate to make a connection that can be relied on. If I know that the patient will come to my ward, I can answer 'Yes, I'll be along to see you tomorrow…' and there may be a visible relaxation in their anxious expression. But if not, I have no choice but to explain, 'No, it won't be me who sees you from now on…but one of the other teams, lung specialists…' Sometimes, if I have spent a good deal of time speaking with them, digging down in important medical or social details, I will add, 'But we will make sure they know all about you…about everything we have discussed…' If it is a crucial fact I will make a point of telling the new team, but more often than not such hand-over of information will occur on paper, in the notes. This requires a clear handwritten entry, a transparent narrative. It is not uncommon for me to see what has been written by the junior doctor accompanying me only to realise that they have not interpreted the patient's words in the same way I have. The emphasis is not quite right. So I re-write it, and leave the ward hoping and expecting that whoever receives that patient will see my note and make sense of it. This is an attempt to maintain the chain of continuity.

I wonder if the psychological distress that derives from uncertainty, not knowing if someone in the machine 'owns' you, if someone is personally invested in your wellbeing, may be sufficient to undo the benefit of technically correct, well timed medical interventions.

Fast track empathy

How do lack of continuity and the diminished feeling of ownership that follows, influence doctors in a way that jeopardises safety? It may hinge on empathy.

Serious illness requires the application of powerful medical interventions. These bring with them the potential for hazard. Recent debate about 'zero harm' culture has crystallised the notion that medicine and its tools can do as much harm as good. To avoid harm staff must be vigilant; they need to keep an eye on the details, spot irregularities, check the blood tests, double check the drug charts, maintain the 'housekeeping' (as it is sometimes called), and anticipate complications. These duties should be automatic, but they are done better if the doctor knows the full story. If they have gained a full appreciation of the patient and their background they will understand better the true impact of those potential harms. Risks and harms can appear abstract, but when they are imagined in the context of the whole person they become tangible, transforming from theoretical 'adverse events' to personal tragedies. A better understanding of those risks may motivate doctors to work harder in ensuring that each job is done properly.

Otherwise they will not be letting down, '…the lady in bed 25, acute kidney injury…', but 'Mrs Jones…she was hoping to get out in time to attend her grand-daughter's wedding this weekend…' Continuity encourages personalisation, personalisation permits the exercise of empathy, and empathy gives our actions relevance.

The challenge for doctors working to shift patterns and caring for patients who arrive to their ward areas on a daily basis, is to learn the practise of empathy in compressed timeframes. This requires active listening, generous emotional investment…energy. But to ensure that connections between patients and doctors are made within the restrictions of the modern hospital environment this has to happen. Otherwise patients will flow through wards without knowing if anyone really 'owned' them, or who that person was. And doctors will float from patient to patient without understanding quite how much trust was being put in them.

Part 4: Assisted dying

The day assisted dying became legal: choices

As a supporter of assisted dying (AD) I ask myself - 'What will I actually do if it becomes legal?' I haven't travelled to Oregon or Washington state to see how it works, nor have I talked to doctors or nurses who are involved, but I think it is important to anticipate one's response. After all, a recent NEJM paper described in a routine, academic, matter of fact way, how a 'Death with dignity' programme was rolled out in a Seattle cancer centre. If AD is legalised in the UK, any doctor who works in the field of cancer or palliative care will be touched by it in some way. The degree of involvement will depend on some of the thought process that I explore in this post.

For those who oppose AD it will be relatively simple – if a patient asks about AD you will make it clear that you do not 'do that'. But it will be necessary to refer the patient on to a colleague who does. To refuse would be to obstruct the patient's access to a legal therapeutic option. There are parallels with abortion here.

What about those who are ambivalent? This is probably the majority. When the day comes, will it be necessary to make a choice, to be an ADer or non-ADer? Will it be necessary to register that preference, for the sake of transparency? Perhaps it will be possible to avoid making that choice for a few months, a year...until a patient asks you to help them. If you are not completely 'anti-' but you have no wish to be involved in assessing them and certifying the terminal nature of their illness, you will again have to refer on. Over time you may be persuaded by the conviction of your patients, and begin to recognise that by referring on and leaving such distasteful tasks to others you are separating yourself from the patient's journey too forcefully. You might conclude that it is cowardly, in a way, to 'wash your hands' of them when the going gets tough and they ask for your signature on the piece of paper, the document, the booklet...whatever it is. You may review your position, and change, finally accepting that 'Yes, quite a few patients have asked me now, AD is a fact of life, why should I make their progress any more difficult than it is already?' Others will remain intellectually neutral, but for good reasons they will continue to maintain clear blue water between their own practice and AD. That will be perfectly understandable. I can foresee many doctors adopting this approach.

And what about doctors like me who instinctively support AD? This is where I get nervous. If, a month after the law is passed, a patient whom I have recently diagnosed with terminal cancer (a common enough event) sits down in my clinic and says, 'When the time comes I want an assisted death. How do I arrange it?' – I will have to do everything in my power to facilitate it. To do otherwise would be hypocritical. So, I might have to decide that I am happy to be one of the signatories, but not so happy to prescribe the fatal dose. Or I might decide to push myself through that discomfort barrier, propelled by a self-imposed reluctance to abdicate my professional responsibility to care for the patient, and volunteer to be physically involved in the prescription and administration of the fatal dose. If I do that I must prepare myself for the experience of being with someone who is *not imminently dying*, who is still independent, in the last hour of their life. I will have to remain strong and unflustered (the last thing they will want to see is a nervous clinician) as they arrive, confirm their identity, take to a bed, gather their family around them, reach for the 'milky drink', and expire. Am I ready for that? Are you?

Assisted dying and The Christian Medical Fellowship: the mercy paradox

In the Assisted Dying (AD) debate the opinion of the Christian Medical Fellowship matters. As an important member of the Care Not Killing Alliance (CNK) it provides solicitors and counsel to oppose changes in the law – the case of Tony Nicklinson being the most recent example. After that disappointing judgment, Dr Andrew Fergusson wrote a guest blog for CMF in which he congratulated the court on their 'compassionate, but dispassionate' approach. CNK, through counsel, intervened in Tony Nicklinson's case, presenting a legalistic argument that stayed away from unpredictable matters of emotion, suffering and frustrated autonomy. This is understandable – what are the courts for, if not to provide an arena in which precedent can be examined, principles tested, and the wisdom of dusty tomes scrutinised in the context of modern medicine? CNK won the day. Tony Nicklinson's application, seeking legal protection for whichever individual volunteered to kill him, was denied. Mr Nicklinson had wanted his case examined in a court of law, and, according to Dr Fergusson,

'That dispassionate discussion has now happened, and disabled people are all the safer for this welcome result.'

Tony Nicklinson's reaction to the judgment was deeply upsetting; his pain was visible and audible. But his determination was undimmed: he refused food – and only the onset of pneumonia, treatment for which he was allowed to refuse, gave him any form of control over his fate. His sadness must have presented a very human, emotional challenge to CMF members who were instrumental in denying him the judgment that he wanted. Without pretending to understand their motives, I would suggest that the theoretical protection of vulnerable individuals from coerced, but legalised, AD was sufficient to salve a sense of guilt. Policies and actions, however unkind they may appear on an individual basis, can be justified if the greater good is served. Indeed Reverend George Pitcher, writing in a Daily Mail blog, stated that TN's suffering was a '…high but necessary price for a civilised society…' This easy calculation, in which individual suffering is counterbalanced by future benefit, troubles me. I want to understand how, in the here and now, a Christian can comfortably engage in a 'dispassionate discussion' while the subject of that discussion man suffers unbearably.

Dr Peter Saunders, CMF Chief Executive, has written the following:

"The current law is clear and right and does not need fixing or further weakening. On the one hand the penalties it holds in reserve act as a powerful deterrent to exploitation and abuse. On the other hand it gives judges some discretion to temper justice

with mercy when sentencing in hard cases. We should not be meddling with it." [http://bit.ly/Rv3gvH]

In the word 'mercy' we see a softening, an appreciation of the suffering that patients and their families are experiencing. He appears to support leniency towards those who facilitate AD, but in 'hard cases' only. The duty to punish an illegal act is tempered by the manifestly unselfish nature of the family's motivation, and the suffering that is visible to all.

This leads to two important questions: how do we define 'hard cases', and does a 'merciful' or lenient approach in such cases represent an implicit acceptance that AD is sometimes right?

There is no spectrum of 'easy' to 'hard' cases in the minds of patients and their families. For them, all are desperately hard. In the eyes of society however, the difficulty of each case is probably related to visibility in the media (the way the story is told) and articulacy of the patient and their family. If a compelling argument is put forward in favour of AD, the case becomes 'hard' in the eyes of the public and the legal/medical professions. They are hard because we see the pain in their eyes, faces and words, and we respond as any human must, with sympathy. The definition of 'hard cases' is therefore subjective, and cannot reasonably be used to decide who should receive mercy. Perhaps we should accept that all cases are hard. But if all cases are hard, shouldn't all families or abettors receive mercy? And if all should receive mercy, the argument for legalisation has been won.

Guidance does exist to help to define which cases should be treated mercifully. Following Deborah Purdy's wish for legal clarification in anticipation of her husband's involvement in her own death (from multiple sclerosis), the courts agreed that the law was not clear. The Director of Public Prosecutions produced a list of factors that would make the prosecution of a someone involved in AD more or less likely. The six factors that reduce the risk of prosecution are:

· The victim had reached a voluntary, clear, settled and informed decision to commit suicide.

· The suspect was wholly motivated by compassion.

· The actions of the suspect, although sufficient to come within the definition of the crime, were of only minor encouragement or assistance.

· The suspect had sought to dissuade the victim from taking the course of action which resulted in his or her suicide.

· The actions of the suspect may be characterised as reluctant encouragement or assistance in the face of a determined wish on the part of the victim to commit suicide.

· The suspect reported the victim's suicide to the police and fully assisted them in their enquiries into the circumstances of the suicide or the attempt and his or her part in providing encouragement or assistance.

Here then is a semi-formalised approach to the definition of 'hard cases'. It is practical, individualised, and a sensible response to the steady trickle of hard cases that nature, in its cruelty, delivers to legal scrutiny. This is the status quo by which CMF have stood so steadfastly. In softening their attitude to suffering they have accepted a compromise. Such laudable *détente* represents a chink in the rather robust CMF armour that was on display during Tony Nicklinson's case. It is, I would argue, an implicit admission that AD happens, and that AD is sometimes right, sometimes the kindest option, sometimes defensible.

I believe that CMF are having it both ways. While opposing the development of a framework in which death can occur legally for those who clearly want it, CMF has accepted that families who help such patients die should be let off. A merciful veneer softens a rigid adherence to principle.

The Tony Nicklinson Judgment

[A shorter version of this appeared in reply to a BMJ blog post at http://t.co/rIQHvTOq on 20th August 2012]

Unfortunately, for those of us who support a change in the law, Tony Nicklinson's case has not advanced the argument very far. I was saddened to see Lord Falconer disagree, albeit sympathetically, with Jane Nicklinson when the two of them were interviewed on Channel 4 news. He did not support TN's campaign. Why?

TN's ambition in seeking legal protection from prosecution for whichever individual agreed to kill him was not representative of the AD movement's aims. There are two reasons for this, as I understand them.

1) He is not terminally ill. AD legislation would be reserved for those who are dying rather than the severely disabled.

2) He requires more than 'assistance' – he is helpless, and needs someone to physically end his life rather than, say, provide a lethal cocktail and arrange it in such a way as to allow him, by his own action, to ingest it.

Hence, AD advocates such as Dignity in Dying and Lord Falconer have not put their full weight behind him. Redefining murder law was always an unlikely result. It is perhaps understandable that AD advocates have kept their powder dry in TN's case, for realistic goals must be set by those wishing to change the law.

The differences between TN and a dying patient care, to my mind, slight, almost semantic. He has suffered what might be described as a social death (a term used in persistent vegetative state literature); he cannot function in society as he would wish. He interacts, yes, and is not as locked in as some have been. But he has decided that his social death should be met by his physical death. Nature will not help him, unless he contracts pneumonia and refuses treatment. He will not starve himself unless he really has to…and that outcome will be a terrible reflection on our society.

So why do I use the word semantic? Because the word being used to describe his possible death is 'murder', whereas the word used to describe the death of say, Diane Pretty (an MS sufferer) is suicide. This is because TN cannot activate a mechanism, but DP can. It is a question of neurological continuity and muscular power. A flick of the finger. An ounce of pressure on a button. The difference between murder and suicide.

There is a huge bioethical problem here. Imagine a patient who is becoming progressively weaker, day by day. Imagine AD has been legalised. Her case has been scrutinised, she has passed each medical and legal hurdle...separate doctors have vouched for her sanity, her consistent approach, the absence of treatable depression, the lack of family coercion...and she succeeds in finding a doctor who will help her. The arrangements are made. A lethal cocktail will be attached to her feeding tube, and when she presses the button a motorised syringe will squeeze the liquid into her stomach. She deteriorates, and loses the power of her fingertips and hands. She cannot activate the machine. She falls outside the legal framework. Now, in a more extreme state of illness and weakness, she is barred from ending her own life. This is a paradox. Because the definition flips from suicide to murder, everything changes.

I understand the stony-faced legal attitude. Law is not there to cater for 'hard cases'. It must protect the majority from abuse. So how do we move on? Most would accept that TN's situation is intolerable, not only for him but for right-thinking, humane observers. How do we allow him to be 'murdered' (a terrible word but to avoid it seems evasive) in a controlled, painless, legal way? There must be a route to individual legislation that does not permit legal precedent by which villainous individuals are allowed to murder sick relatives and then argue that it was their wish to be killed. The law cannot be that blunt.

Part 5: Medical error

Memory failure after medical error: the building blocks of experience

There is a contradiction in medicine that has always interested me – the need to form a complete psycho-social picture of each individual patient (aiding empathy) *versus* the need to depersonalise, categorise and store their medical story (thus adding to experience). When things go wrong, this tension results in a paradoxical lack of humanity.

Example: a junior doctor, two years qualified, makes a mistake. She writes the wrong antibiotic up on a Friday afternoon, having failed to check the result of cultures that were taken three days before. The bacteria causing the infection is not sensitive to the antibiotic that she prescribes. The patient deteriorates. The doctor recognises and regrets her error, watches the patient and his family, learns all that there is to know about his life and background. He dies two weeks later (his death the result of multiple diseases, not just her action). She is devastated. For days and weeks she reflects on her mistake. A vivid image of the family keeps entering her mind, as do their words, when they asked how a simple urine infection could make someone this ill. Moreover she checks the computer assiduously before prescribing antibotics from then on.

Twelve years later she is asked to deliver an induction lecture to new doctors. She emphasises how important it is that they check each result for themselves, take nothing for granted…watch the details. She is a very careful doctor, always was really, except for that one slip which happened early on. She drives home…and casts her mind back to the moment she learned that her patient had grown worse over the weekend, due, in part, to her brief incompetence. She finds that she cannot remember his name. She cannot form a picture of his face in her mind's eye. The family…how many were there? The man has gone…only the error, and the lesson that grew out that error, remains. The individual has been subsumed by history, by a thousand other patients with a thousand different problems.

We cannot be expected to remember every patient, of course. But those who made the greatest impressions on us might, you would think, linger on in our memories. Indeed they do, but mainly in the form of salient facts – the features and factors that made them special, be they medical, situational, or personal. Their memory survives as a construct that exists only in relation to the effect it had on you, the doctor, rather than the self-contained, individual and tragic story that the patient's demise truly signified in their world…a world that you, as their doctor, were never really a party to.

It is a subtle and rather esoteric observation, I admit it, but for me it feeds into a larger question. How do doctors 'process' the memories of patients who once presented a great medical or personal challenge?

A mature doctor will have been buffeted and battered by numerous 'bad outcomes'. That cold phrase describes unexpected injury, suffering or death of patients related to decisions or treatments ministered by us, their doctors. Those outcomes may have been inevitable, but the fact that they occurred after we saw them and gave advice forms a link in our mind. Was it something I did? Should I have made a different decision? Was I wrong? And if I was wrong, what will I do differently next time? A lesson is learnt, and each little shock, each piece of bad news, adds to the pattern of experience that forms the value of a good doctor. We carry those lessons around with us, making sure that next time we encounter a similar situation we do not make the same mistake. We get better, and feel more confident. The price – a series of personal tragedies that become smaller and smaller in our memory as time passes. All but the most harrowing (or perhaps those that resulted in sharp criticism or professional censure) lose their emotional edge. We recall the events in abstract – 'I did this, this happened, he died, I felt awful…oh yes, I don't recommend it, don't ever do that…' – but we are no longer visibly damaged. In fact we are wiser and stronger, and at some level perhaps we are grateful for having been through it.

My point is that the lifelong process of learning that *is* a medical career requires us to find a way to live through these setbacks and make something positive out of them. To do this doctors must strip those memories of the very qualities that made them so powerful in the first place…the patients' suffering and the impact this had on those around them. The lesson learnt is usually one of process, data interpretation, practical technique or communication…whatever it is it is something to do with the doctor. It is the doctor who is the constant, whereas the patient, even though their specific needs and problems formed the basis of the risk, is one of many who will cross that doctor's path.

So is all this a problem? It is if we become too good at the process of assimilation and are tempted to put each mistake 'down to experience' too soon. It is if we do not dwell sufficiently on the impact of mistakes that, from a medical point of view, were purely 'technical'. It is if we immediately compartmentalise those errors, surrounding (or hiding) them in hastily erected walls of rationalisation, forensic examination and (instinctive) defensiveness, thereby underplaying their social significance. I wonder if such post-hoc failures of imagination and empathy that can lead to a lack of candour. When errors are immediately assessed in relation to the system that caused them rather than the social unit, the family, that was most directly affected by them, we are in effect turning away from the pain and settling our gaze on our own concerns. That has to happen of course, if weaknesses in the system are to be addressed, but the timing and the emphasis have to be right.

Personally, as a doctor who has been blown off course as frequently as any other, I think depersonalisation and abstraction are vital. They are not particularly warm or human traits, but they are understandable. The process of learning from experience must be the same for doctors as it is for any other professional, and the same need to filter, discard and retain the 'essence' of each incident applies. The difference, for doctors, is that the extraneous matter is often deep emotion and human pain.

A 'Never Event' and the chain of blame

This is an example of worst case scenario thinking. It is an entirely fictional case. I have used the same approach that I use in my medical fiction, working out how, within the boundaries of plausibility afforded by standard clinical processes and environments, a particular error might occur. Perhaps this accident happened somewhere, sometime…I don't know.

This exercise in imagination is intended to show how difficult it is determine where blame lies. Few medical mistakes, in my experience, occur because one person made one mistake. There is often a 'series of unfortunate events', each one of which could, perhaps should, have been recognised and reversed before the next occurred. As I read about the 'duty of candour' in the Francis report on Mid-Staffs, and read about Jeremy Hunt's response to it on behalf of the government, I reflected that each time a patient is harmed it will become necessary for hospital Trusts to make a judgement as to whether the incident requires a patient or family to be contacted (whether or not they have complained). It is clear now that there will be no legal compunction for individual healthcare professionals to admit to and communicate these errors, but organisations as a whole (embodied by 'the board') will have to recognise and act on that duty. It is not clear to me how this will work. Organisations are collections of individuals, and for the truth about avoidable harms to rise to the top those involved on the shop floor will have to be honest and forthcoming.

I wondered how individuals would respond in a 'harm' situation. I tried to imagined a scenario that should *never* happen, but did. Never Events are medical mistakes that the NHS Litigation Authority (NHSLA) have deemed avoidable and, to be blunt, indefensible. They are, *'serious, largely preventable patient safety incidents that should not occur if the available preventative measures have been implemented.'* Never Events are reported annually, and spikes in their frequency tend to be picked up by the press (as in Derriford, Plymouth in March 2013).

One Never Event is when liquid food is poured down a nasogastric feeding tube (NGT) that has been accidentally inserted into a lung. If food is dripped into such a misplaced tube the patient will literally begin to drown, and the consequences of this range from becoming transiently short of oxygen, to developing pneumonia, requiring mechanical ventilation or dying. Hospitals have protocols that are designed to ensure that this never happens, and the NHSLA has published algorithms to minimise the risk.

Here then is a reconstruction of how this Never Event might happen; as you read it, ask yourself who is to blame and how it might be communicated to the family.

-/-

The date was 2rd February 2013 (a Saturday).

Mr Mohammad Ghazi was 78 years old, and had been admitted one week previously with a stroke which affected his ability to swallow. He was fed via a NGT, but on two previous occasions he had accidentally dislodged the tube.

Dr Martin Simpson didn't know Mr Ghazi. He was asked to get involved at 5.30pm on the Saturday in question. The nurse in charge of the ward, Susan, called him to report that Mr Ghazi had pulled out his latest NG tube in the morning, and that she had inserted another at 3pm. However she could not get a reliable pH (gastric acidity) reading from the aspirate, which she attributed to him having residual feed in the stomach and the fact he was on high dose acid suppressants. Without the acidity test she could not confirm that the tube was actually in the stomach, and protocol dictated that a chest x-xray (CXR) was required. Martin agreed to arrange the CXR and promised to look at it before he finished his shift at 9pm. He asked Susan to bleep him when the x-ray had been done; he was going to be busy clerking new patients in A&E, as the registrar had requested that he help the admitting team during the traditional early evening rush. Martin sent an electronic x-ray request through and forgot about it. Someone would let him know when the x-ray was ready.

At 8.30 pm Susan walked onto the ward having popped out to pick up a drug from pharmacy for another patient. She held the door open for the porter who was bringing Mr Ghazi back from the x-ray department. She helped the porter wheel Mr Ghazi's bed into the empty bay and, noting the time, went to bleep Martin. He answered promptly, logged on to the x-ray programme on a computer in A&E, scanned along the list of Mr Ghazi's x-rays, clicked onto the one dated 3/2/2013 and saw that the tube position was perfect. The tip of the tube lay well below the diaphragm, it crossed the edge of the main airway, it was definitely in the stomach. He called the ward, Susan answered, and Martin confirmed that he was happy for her to commence the feed that night. Martin left at 9.30pm. Susan left at 10pm, leaving it to the next shift to turn the feed on.

At 11pm the ward sister on the night shift, Mary, answered the phone. It was the x-ray department, ringing to see if Mr Ghazi was available to come for his x-ray. Mary answered that he had already had it. No, said the radiographer, the request hadn't been checked off. 'Why was in he taken down to the department earlier then?' asked Mary. The radiographer checked the system – oh yes, that had been for an ultrasound which had been booked a couple of days ago; the on-call radiologist had decided to do it that evening in order to clear the backlog. He hadn't yet had the x-ray for the new NG tube.

Mary ran to the bedside. Liquid food was being dripped into the tube. Mr Ghazi was breathing badly. She stopped the feed immediately and called the medical team. The night doctor came to the ward and logged onto the x-ray programme. The x-ray that Martin had looked at was the wrong one – the right date, but the wrong time, taken in the very early hours of the *same day* to check the *previous* NG tube, the one that had been removed.

Mr Ghazi developed pneumonia, deteriorated and died a week later.

Investigation – assumptions and facts

The investigation showed that Martin had indeed looked at the wrong x-ray, and that the right x-ray had never been done. Susan was mistaken in telling Martin that the x-ray had been done – when she saw Mr Ghazi returning to the ward with the porter she had *assumed*, erroneously, that he had just had his x-ray. That assumption went unchallenged, and when Martin saw that an x-ray had been performed on the relevant date he *assumed* this was the new one. He did not check the time.

When the x-ray was eventually performed it showed that the new NG tube was in the right lung, and the lung was already turning white, filling with liquid feed.

Testimonies

Susan: I saw him being wheeled in. It was natural to assume he was coming back from his chest x-ray. I didn't even know he was booked for an ultrasound. He had come to our ward the day before, it must have been booked when he was on the other ward. The timing fitted. Do I think what happened is my fault? No, actually. It wasn't me who checked the x-ray…

Martin: I'd never met him. I didn't know him, didn't know he'd had an NG tube down just the day before, that it had been x-rayed overnight, at 2 in the morning! Susan…and I'm not blaming her…told me that he had come back from his x-ray. I saw on the computer that there was an x-ray taken on the day in question, it looked fine. Why didn't I check the time? I can make excuses…I was rushing, but aren't we all, all the time. I was clerking, when actually I was supposed to be on ward cover…but if I'd been doing that I would have been just a busy probably. You know, I can't see how this could have been avoided. Not unless there was some way of linking the x-ray to the specific NG tube insertion. How could you do that?

Susan: His son came in, sat with him as he died. We didn't send him to intensive care, he would never have survived on a ventilator. I explained how food had got into his lung, and he didn't ask me how, or why… he didn't assume a mistake had been made. And it wasn't the right time to go into all the details then and there. He had to have some time to grieve…I think that's reasonable. We didn't hide anything.

Mary: I felt awful. I set up the feed pump. As soon as I turned it on the feed began to drip into his lung. I did that, I can't get away from that. But should I, personally, have checked the tube was correctly sited? I don't think so. I'm not trained to look at x-rays. Martin, the doctor, told me it was fine. I can't do more than that…can I?

Martin: Because he wasn't actually my patient I didn't find out until the following Wednesday. The registrar on the stroke team came to find me, and let me know. She told me there was bound to be a complaint. I asked her straight away if the family had been told. I volunteered to tell them…but she said it would wait, and that their team would deal with it. But she did advise me to write everything down, all the details, in case I ended up giving evidence to the coroner. I went home and typed up a narrative… I still have it.

The clinical director: The simplest, harshest analysis is that Martin was negligent in not confirming that the x-ray he saw related to the new NG tube. If he had taken note of the time on the screen he would have realised immediately. But I'm sympathetic to his explanation. There was duplication. Two x-rays requested in a short period of time, less than 24 hours. Perhaps, just as we highlight and take special precautions if there are two patients with the same surname on a ward, we should highlight if two tests are arranged for the same patient…to ensure the right one is looked at. This terrible event has exposed a weakness in the system. I have never heard this happen before, anywhere. So it's hard to say to the family, yes, we made a terrible mistake and did badly by your husband and father…we did, of course, but I cannot see where we could have done better on the night in question. The mistake was there waiting to be made, all the time. It could have been anyone who made it. We now need to look at ways of making sure it never happens again.

The Board (a representative): We were all agreed, we needed to tell the family. By the time we discussed it the initial investigations had been completed, and it became clear that the family had no idea that a mistake had been made. That made it more difficult than if they had been told straight away. It came as a complete and utter surprise to them, to the son anyway…he was the main contact. But even then there was no anger. It won't always be like that obviously…but this family were philosophical, and took the view, very reasonably, that medical interventions come with inherent risks. We do not necessarily take that view – feeding through a tube should not be risky. That's why it's a 'never event'. It is avoidable.

The family (his son): The Trust were candid with us. They called me, invited me in for an interview, and the consultant explained what had happened. Although I had never heard of Never Events, I realised once they admitted to us that it was food in the lung that killed him that this should never have happened. It's basic. But I read their investigation, and I can't see who or what to blame. The poor guy who saw the wrong x-ray, his is probably the greatest responsibility. But if I blame anyone I blame the Trust…did it go over how crucial it is to double check the time, did it train its junior doctors for that situation? Perhaps they should train nurses to read these x-rays, I don't know. You might think that's an overreaction, but this was supposed to be a 'never' event…and it happened. By definition therefore, inadequate preparations had been made. They hadn't thought it through…not until my father died.

Fatal error: a doctor deals with the harm she did

Junior doctors make mistakes, and how they deal with those mistakes is of crucial importance. In this dialogue I explore the psychological reaction and coping mechanisms of a Foundation Year doctor who has made a drug error, contributing to the death of a patient. She speaks with her registrar, who has been though a similar experience. As usual, it is fictional, but based on my observations of myself and others since qualifying.

It is worth considering how common drug errors are. Dean et al, in their BMJ paper 'Prescribing errors in hospital inpatients: their incidence and clinical significance' (2002) found during a 4 week period, which involved about 36,200 medication orders, that,

'a prescribing error was identified in 1.5%. A potentially serious error occurred in 0.4%. Most of the errors (54%) were associated with choice of dose.'

Finlay and Ross, in a BMJ editorial 'Medication errors caused by juniors' (2008), wrote,

'Preventable medication errors account for 10-20% of adverse events in patients admitted to hospital... The situation is similar in Australia and the US—medication errors occur in about 1-2% of

patients admitted to hospital, resulting in around 7000 deaths a year in the US alone.'

The public are well aware of the potential for harm, not necessarily related to medications, with articles such as this in the Evening Standard (2002), which said:

'Alarming failures in the education and training of junior doctors could be contributing to the thousands of medical errors, including hundreds of deaths, which occur in hospitals every year…'

The consequences of error are never underestimated by doctors. But the Francis report, in emphasising the duty of candour in admitting mistakes to patients and families, has focussed attention of the subject. It is vital that doctors who make mistakes can admit to them, but be supported while they work through the implications. If there is need for re-training, so be it. If errors seem to be repeated, or the doctor appears unable to accept a need to improve, then certainly their career choice will need to be reconsidered. For the majority of doctors who make a mistake however, it will be an isolated or very infrequent event. The way they deal with it requires some examination. This is how one such doctor deals with it.

Scene: a quiet corner in the doctors' mess.

An FY1 (Foundation Year doctor, in her first year of employment since qualifying) and her registrar.

Registrar: What happened?

FY1: I made a mistake. A really bad one. Somebody died.

I heard about it. How are you doing?

Awful. I feel awful.

Are you worried? About your career?

Yes, well no, not about being in trouble so much. I know there will be an investigation, but one of my friends did something similar last year...

What happened to him?

He had to go on a course, pharmacology and prescribing, and he had to be observed doing drug charts for 6 weeks. But he got through it.

I can't guarantee it'll be that straightforward this time, but you're right, I don't see why you should be struck off or anything like that. Not for a one off error. The irony is, however many courses you go on, after this you will never prescribe a drug again without being one hundred percent sure that the dose is right. You'll be paranoid, but you'll be safer than most of your mates.

I don't want to prescribe anything again. I feel sick whenever I see a drug chart now. I'm avoiding writing any prescriptions.

That's not good. We can't have you not functioning properly. But it will get easier, I promise.

You've had this experience?

Every single doctor you ever meet will have had this experience. Any doctor working in acute medicine will know what it feel like to have done harm.

And how did you cope?

You have to find a way through it. You have to be able to see through it, to the other side. You know you're going to be a doctor, working for years and years probably, so you have to put it into perspective. But at the same time you can't ignore the importance of it.

That's what's worrying me. I can't see myself doing this for ever. It's too painful, having experiences like this. I know, when I think about it, that Mr _ would be alive, now, if I hadn't written that prescription. Or if I had double checked the dose. He was due to go home in two days! I know that mistakes often have multiple reasons behind them, system errors, but in this case it was me, just me. I actually remember writing it, the word, the number. I can't handle that, not again.

You are handling it now, in a way. You're here, at work, not at home sick, you're talking about it. You're finding a way through it.

But I don't want to be here. You know what I want? I want to be home with my Mum and Dad.

That's natural. It's a need for security, for comfort. It's a response to acute stress.

And I keep thinking about dropping out. I have this fantasy of running a book shop, just sitting there, no stress. I walked past one of the cleaners this morning, and I was jealous. I wanted to do her job. No stress. No complications. Simple tasks…

I know what you're saying, but it's not real. That cleaner probably has more stress in her life, more persistently, than you do. You are lucky, you have an amazingly satisfying job. You will always be needed, there will always be patients that need to see you. You have been trained to do that job, and I know that fundamentally you enjoy it! I've seen you at work remember. You are enthusiastic and genuinely interested. I've got no doubt that you'll be fine.

They won't be coming to see me! If I'm not there, there will be another doctor in my place. I'm not indispensible.

Of course. Nobody is. But you have the potential to be very good and to be important to your patients, and to the doctors that you in

turn will train. The way I think is this, and I know it sounds harsh –
but you have a responsibility to get over this setback.

Mr_ isn't going to get over this setback, is he?

That's not the way to think about it.

Why? Is my career more important than him?

Of course not. And his death will receive it's due attention, we will
all look at ourselves. Did we train you properly? Was the system
for checking prescriptions working? Were the side effects
recognised? His death will not just go unremarked. We will, we
have, apologised to his family. The coroner will undoubtedly
examine the sequence of events. It's not going to trivialised or
brushed under the carpet. But is it right that the mistake should
result in a potentially excellent doctor leaving medicine? No, it
isn't. There would be no doctors left!

I feel really uncomfortable with this. It does feel as though we are
belittling his memory, focussing on my future.

When I was in your position, years ago, I just kept it all in, didn't
talk about it. Perhaps there's something to be said for that.

I'm a talker I'm afraid. I have to talk. Do you mind?

No, of course not. Look, this is how it goes. Or how it went for me.
I made a mistake, it doesn't matter what exactly. A patient died. I

hated medicine. I didn't want to come in. I avoided similar situations, just like you have been doing. And then, you know what happened?

What?

Life happened, that's what. By which I mean, the sun rose and the sun set, shifts came and went, patients arrived that needed to be seen, and they kept coming, and I had to see them and treat them. There was no option. And three weeks later I looked back, and thought – shit, I've seen hundreds of patients since I made that mistake, and nothing bad has happened. I felt safe again, in myself. I felt like a safe doctor. That's how it went for me.

Riding a bike.

Kind of. You have the skills and the knowledge. You have identified something about yourself through this error...the fact that your memory for drug doses is not perfect, and you have learnt from it. Depending on the policy of this trust, which I don't know, you may have to do some 'remedial' course or programme, and if that's the case, fine, accept it. Penance. But in three weeks, I promise you, the pain you feel now will be a mental bruise. You'll never forget it, but it will fade.

Easy as that.

Not easy. Because it will happen again. You can't have a career in medicine, especially a practical specialty, or surgery, if you're that way inclined, and not cause harm occasionally. Every invasive procedure has a complication rate, by their very nature. The chance that you will be the one who *never* has a complication is infinitesimal. So you have to find a way to deal with it. It's going to happen. This is your first time. Your colleagues may experience it this year, next year, in three years time. Perhaps it's good to go through it now, I don't know. How are you feeling?

Just as bad.

I can't change that. But time will.

Why Michael didn't blow the whistle: pub scene

In this imagined scene I explore the reasons why junior doctors rarely blow the whistle on poorly performing senior colleagues. I have not been in this situation, and the words I place in the mouths and minds of my protagonists are based on supposition. Of course, real whistleblowers would be able to shed a more penetrating light on this dilemma. Their descriptions would have far more validity. But many junior doctors will have observed poor practice, and they will have considered the question – should I tell somebody? Perhaps this post goes some way to explaining why they hardly ever do.

Readers of this blog will know my methods – I take the true essence of a problem and enlarge it in my imagination. I do not pretend to justify actions or omissions here. It is merely an attempt to explain how people think.

oOo

A junior doctor called Michael observes that his consultant, Doctor G, has made what he believes is the wrong diagnosis on three separate occasions. Michael thinks he has detected a pattern of medical inadequacy. The first time, Dr G failed to detect or interpret the signs of early septic shock on a post-take ward round. Two hours later the patient was in intensive care, on quadruple strength noraderenaline, having been transferred in a state of peri-arrest. On the second occasion an elderly patient with leg weakness was assumed to be 'off legs' due to a urine infection, but the following day, after the man had been examined more thoroughly, a spinal cord tumour was found on an MRI scan. He was rushed to a neurosurgical unit for emergency decompressive surgery. And on the third occasion a patient with liver cirrhosis was, in the view of the junior doctor, written off without serious consideration being given to organ support and transfer to the intensive care unit.

Michael brooded on these examples. One evening he begins to moan about Doctor G in the pub. He relates the three incidents. His friend, another doctor, nods with common feeling. Michael realises at once that this consultant had an established reputation, a bad one, among other juniors .

"So what has been done about it?" he asks.

"The guy's been there for years, he'll be retiring in another couple." says his friend.

"So?"

"He trained in a different era. Half the diseases and treatments that we see now he didn't even learn about."

"That's no excuse."

"What do you expect the trust to do?"

"Take him off the rota. Patients are being exposed to him every week."

"And what would that cost? They'd have to employ another consultant."

"Does it matter?"

"No, of course not. But can you prove that he has actually caused a patient to suffer or die."

"Well we have just discussed cases where that has obviously happened. I can't believe nobody has ever said anything."

"So are you going to do it? Whistleblow?"

"I'm tempted to. Who should I talk to?"

"You're educational supervisor. That's who I would go to. Is he friendly, your supervisor?"

"She's a she. A surgeon. I'm not sure she would have a strong opinion on the medical detail."

"It doesn't matter. She doesn't have to. She just has to acknowledge your concern. She'll have an obligation to go up the chain. What about the GMC?"

"What will they do?"

"I've heard there's a hotline they're setting up."

"You know what I think would happen if I told them?"

"What?"

"I think it would ruin my life."

"Why?"

"Because for the rest of my time here I would be thinking about what was going to happen."

"In what way?"

"Well…I'm sure they would be discrete, but they would need evidence from me. I would have to provide some reports or they would have to come down and find them. That would become the focus of my life. Makes me feel ill thinking about it."

"We had something like this on the ethics station in our exam.   If   there was a real, imminent risk of patient safety the answer was easy. You have to remove the doctor from the clinical environment."

"Yes, but that was for doctors on drugs, or drunk ."

"What's the difference? A danger is a danger. If you really think he's a danger then you should go to someone. The medical director or something like that?"

"Didn't you work out with them a while back? Didn't you notice anything?"

"Yes, I thought he was crap."

"So did you go and speak to anybody?"

"No. He wasn't *that* crap."

"But now you know, having spoken to me, that he is *that* crap. We agree. I'm sure if there were a few others in here we'd all agree. Shouldn't we all do something about it?"

There is a silence. What is going through their minds?

Perhaps this: it was not clear to either that Doctor G was a genuine danger. For prior to their arrival in the trust, just two and half months ago, this doctor had been employed for over 20 years without serious complaint. So why should it come to them, these young doctors at the beginning of their careers, to raise the alarm? Surely, if no-one else had detected his deficiencies it was more likely that *they* were wrong. Perhaps their inexperience had led them to misinterpret the things they had witnessed. There was more to medical decision making than they currently understood. It was more subtle than right or wrong...

And after all, did those patients *really* suffer more because of Doctor G's decisions? The man with septic shock recovered eventually. The liver patient, a dyed in the wool alcoholic, was always going to die anyway. The intensive care docs were bound to have said no. And the patient with the spinal cord tumour was making a slow recovery; those extra hours without a diagnosis had not rendered him permanently paralysed. You could argue that it was responsibility of the A&E staff, or the admitting medical registrar, to examine him more thoroughly and detect the tell-tale sensory level. Can you expect consultants, who see each patient for ten minutes after they have already been the hospital for up to twelve hours already, to make every diagnosis, to make no errors? And hadn't the consultant seen another 15 patients on that post a ward round, making the right diagnosis and the right decision for the overwhelming majority?

Michael begins to feel better, more settled. The dangers, to himself, melt away a little. He isn't betraying his patients' trust by avoiding the confrontation. Doctor G is different. He has strengths… and weaknesses. Clinically suspect, perhaps, but part of the old guard. And, when it comes down to it, Michael is pretty sure he does a lot more good than harm in the hospital.

"Where do you rotate to next?" asks Michael's friend.

"Ortho."

"Life might be a bit more straightforward there."

"I know it will."

"Two weeks."

"Head down mate."

Part 6: Care towards the end of life and resuscitation

Not For This and Not For that: emphasising the positive in care for the elderly

It is a sad truth that we sometimes spend as much time deciding what *not* to do when treating elderly patients as we do determining what options are appropriate. The early part of each admission is straightforward enough – we take a history, perform an examination, form a list of possible diagnoses and initiate treatment of some sort. But as we walk away at the end of the day, part of our duty is to consider what will happen if the patient deteriorates. If, in the middle of the night, or over the weekend, they suffer some sort of collapse – what instructions should we leave?

In most cases we do not need to leave specific instructions, because the hospital is set up to deal with such emergencies. The patient's worsening condition will be identified by a nurse, the on call team will be bleeped (perhaps a 'MET'* call will be put out), resuscitative measures will be taken and they may even be transferred to the high dependency or intensive care unit. If their heart stops they will undergo cardio-pulmonary resuscitation (CPR). That is the default. For many though, such a sequence of events will prove disastrous.

The reasons why very elderly or already frail patients should not undergo resuscitation have been rehearsed on this blog before, but many of those arguments apply to ICU admission too. The potential benefits are so slight that the definite burdens (such as prolonged ventilation, tracheostomy insertion, connection to a dialysis machine via central venous catheters, critical care neuropathy) cannot be justified. So, it is necessary to determine in advance whether those options are offered.

This is reasonably straightforward if the patient is alert and understands the issues. Unfortunately, a large proportion of acutely unwell elderly patients do not have the capacity to engage in such a conversation when they arrive in hospital. We therefore turn to the family, and by combining what we learn about their pre-existing wishes with what we anticipate are the possible benefits of organ support, we set 'ceilings of treatment'. We try to work out what the patient would want if they could talk to us clearly. We make an informed guess, then we write in the notes phrases such as:

Not for ICU

Not for MET

Not for escalation

Ward based care only

Not for filtration

Not for NG tube

Not for NIV**

Not for ventilation, for NIV only…

Not for this, not for that. A typical ward round or on-call shift might require many such decisions, and it can feel overwhelmingly negative. Doctors are trained to treat actively, but increasingly, as the population ages and more and more patients are admitted to hospital toward the end of the expected human life span, they have to be protect them from the full gamut of invasive medical procedures. And the less information they have about the patient's preferences, the greater the weight of responsibility in setting those 'ceilings'.

How then to change the emphasis and accentuate the positive, focus on what we can do, and not what we cannot?

It's all about anticipation. I am always amazed when patients in their nineties, or their families, express surprise when I bring up the possibility that they might die. It seems never to have crossed their minds! This natural reluctance to consider death has been challenged. Dying Matters (a coalition led by the National Council for Palliative Care) highlights that,

81% of people have not written down any preferences around their own death

Nearly two thirds (63%) of us would prefer to die at home, yet of the 500,000 people who die each year in England, 53% die in hospital.

They request that people consider,

The type of care you would like towards the end of your life

Where you would like to die

Whether you have any particular worries you would like to discuss about being ill and dying

Whether you want to be resuscitated or not

'It's OK to die', an organisation in the United States set up by Monica Williams Murphy MD, advocates a similar set questions. Imagine if every patient came into hospital with this information. No more guess work. No more stressed families trying to explain what their elderly relative would have wanted, feeling the weight of responsibility even when reassured that they are not being asked to make 'life or death decisions'.

Engaging in these questions may not be natural. Those with manifestly terminal conditions may be drawn into such discussions by their families, palliative care teams or general practitioners (GPs, family doctors), but those who are in their ninth and tenth decades without end stage disease are not necessarily going to dwell on their mortality. It falls to their GPs to initiate the discussion.

The concept of the Advance Care Plan (ACP) is well established, albeit in the context of life limiting conditions. The document 'Advance Care Planning: A Guide for Health and Social Care Staff' specifies that,

The difference between ACP and care planning more generally is that the process of ACP will usually take place in the context of an anticipated deterioration in the individual's condition in the future, with attendant loss of capacity to make decisions and/or ability to communicate wishes to others.

It might seem then ACPs are not intended for people in a stable condition who are in no imminent danger of deteriorating. The document does however include this common, 'non-terminal' example scenario:

Mrs Carter – An 81 year old lady with COPD, heart failure, osteoarthritis and increasing forgetfulness, who lives alone. She fractured her hip after a fall, eats a poor diet and finds mobility difficult. She wishes to stay at home but is increasingly unable to cope alone and appears to be 'skating on thin ice'.

Perhaps then it is not unreasonable to introduce the idea of an ACP to people with common cardio-respiratory problems that do not seem 'life-limiting' in the most obvious sense.

The same document is explicit that:

If an advance decision includes refusal of life sustaining treatment, it must be in writing, signed and witnessed and include the statement 'even if life is at risk'

And warns that it,

Only comes in effect if the treatment and circumstances are those specifically identified in the advance decision

These stipulations make ACPs less workable in primary care or general medicine. How can a person be expected to anticipate specific circumstances? How will they know, in advance, what the burden of those life sustaining treatments will be, in relation to the possible benefits. Again, the emphasis is on the negative. Wouldn't it be more helpful to know what they *do* want, what their ultimate goals are. For instance, 'to be able to look after myself when I get home, feed myself, to interact with my grandchildren...' These goals may preclude extended life preserving treatment that can be reliably predicted to result in chronic debilitation or loss of independence. They may be better suited to a 'Preferred Priorities of Care' statement. In reality, I suspect the term ACP is used in a more general way than intended.

150

Do ACPs work? There is some evidence. A study by Karen M Detering et al (BMJ 2009) randomised 154 of 309 mentally competent octogenarian in-patients to the make an ACP, and found,

Of the 56 patients who died by six months, end of life wishes were much more likely to be known and followed in the intervention group (25/29, 86%) compared with the control group (8/27, 30%; P<0.001).

In the intervention group, family members of patients who died had significantly less stress (intervention 5, control 15; P<0.001), anxiety (intervention 0, control 3; P=0.02), and depression (intervention 0, control 5; P=0.002) than those of the control patients.

A proactive approach to ACP (or equivalent) is not without risk. As part of the National End of Life Care Strategy GPs were encouraged to identify those under their care who were predicted to die in the next twelve months, and to make a list. Some parts of the press did not take this well;

Thousands of patients have already been placed on 'death registers' which single them out to be allowed to die in comfort rather than be given life-saving treatment in hospital, it emerged last night.

151

Nearly 3,000 doctors have promised to draw up a list of patients they believe are likely to die within a year, Department of Health figures showed yesterday.

As part of an unpublicised campaign endorsed by ministers, GPs have been encouraged to make lists – officially known as End of Life Care Registers – of people they believe are going to die soon and should be helped to do so in comfort. (Daily Mail, 18th October 2012)

The subject became entangled with the Liverpool Care Pathway controversy. I don't know if the registers have continued to be compiled. The taboo of death remains strong. But the idea is sound. Dying Matters have promoted the 'Find your 1%' approach. They request that GPs ask themselves,

"Would I be surprised if this person were to die in the next 12 months?"

Apparently,

...this simple question is accurate seven times out of ten.

They emphasise some general indicators of likely death within 12 months:

- Limited self-care and interest in life: in bed or a chair more than 50% of their time.

- Breathless at rest or on minimal exertion

- Progressive weight loss (>10% over last six months).

- History of recurring or persistent infections and/or pressure ulcers.

The GMC too recognises the importance of being forward about end of life care planning. Its <u>End of Life Care booklet</u> includes this:

If a patient in your care has a condition that will impair their capacity as it progresses, or is otherwise facing a situation in which loss or impairment of capacity is a foreseeable possibility, you should encourage them to think about what they might want for themselves should this happen, and to discuss their wishes and concerns with you and the healthcare team.

Areas for discussion include:

– the patient's wishes, preferences or fears in relation to their future treatment and care

– interventions which may be considered or undertaken in an emergency, such as cardiopulmonary resuscitation (CPR), when it may be helpful to make decisions in advance

– the patient's preferred place of care (and how this may affect the treatment options available)

These initiatives and guidelines are fine, but harder to achieve than they are to promote. Talking about death is never easy (for families or doctors), and it is still more common than not for patients to be admitted with no evidence, verbal or written, of their fears, priorities or goals. It falls on doctors and nurses whom the patients have never met to introduce the subject and explore those issues…or, when mental capacity has been lost, to gather clues from the family who may not have had those conversation either. Until this changes it will remain a sad part of our role to gauge how far each patient should be escalated, hoping always that our judgment is correct.

Notes

* MET score – medical emergency team; most hospitals now have an 'early warning' system for deteriorating patients, whereby nurses can summon the on-call team if there are dangerous blood pressure, pulse rate or respiratory changes.

** NIV = non-invasive ventilation; a tight mask is applied to the face to improve lung function, effective but often quite unpleasant as the patient is awake

Complaint: a grieving son meets the consultant who signed a DNAR form without discussion

This dialogue is part of a continuing examination into the interactions that occur when doctors and families meet at the end of life. The way that these two parties react to death, the emotions that they project and the decisions they make, must derive from the same understanding of the patient's needs if conflict is to be avoided. Sadly that is not always the case, and readers of this blog may be aware of cases where disagreement has led to complaint, and sometimes to court.

In this scenario, an 79 year old woman was admitted to hospital with pneumonia. The medical team recognized that she was deteriorating quickly, and that resuscitation would not be effective. An attempt was made to contact her next of kin, a 54 year old son, by telephone, but there was no answer machine. He lived 200 miles away, although two other children lived closer. She died 18 hours after admission, and no attempt was made to resuscitate her. Following a complaint, that son has arranged to meet the consultant in charge of his mother's care.

Of the many factors that contribute to a lack of assiduity in making sure that discussions about resuscitation occur, an important one, I feel, is what I call the 'normalisation of death'. Here, the relative comes to a similar conclusion, and challenges the consultant.

The son (S) sits in an office with the medical consultant (C), a senior nurse and a member of the PALS team. Only S and C speak.

———

C: Thank you for coming.

S: I just want to know why you made that decision without asking us, her family. I was listed as next of kin.

C: Of course we need to discuss why it was decided that your mother should not be resuscitated without your involvement, but it is very important for you to realise that the decision was not made lightly. Her death was felt to be inevitable. We thought that there was absolutely no hope of recovery. We always try to discuss those decisions with relatives but sometimes it is just not possible.

S: But how could you make that decision to let her die without asking us? She would not have wanted you to give up so easily. We would have told you that.

C: It was not a matter of 'letting her die'. We knew that she was likely to die despite everything that we were doing, and that resuscitation would not have worked. So yes, we did permit her to die, because we saw the signs that this was inevitable. We never had a chance of stopping it happening. She was not deprived of a meaningful opportunity to survive…in our opinion.

S: But she never had a chance without it. She would have wanted you to try – your interpretation of meaningful is…*your* interpretation. What of hers or ours?

C: Well, if she understood the very tiny chance of success, I don't think she would have wanted us to resuscitate.

S: How can you say that? You didn't know her. She never gave up on anything. However small the chance of success, she pursued it, in all areas of her life.

C: I'm sure she did. I definitely got that impression from her and from the background history that we learned about her. But we are talking about a different sort of chance here. The risks in making a decision on this small chance were probably more grave than those she was used to in other areas of her life. The risk was definite harm and suffering. In fact it wasn't a risk…it was a certainty.

S: Still, it was not up to you to make that decision. It was not your body or your mother. We should have been involved. And we know that you are required to involve us. It's in all of the regulations and professional guidelines.

C: You are right, it is. But those guidelines cannot apply to every single situation. And this was a special situation. She was deteriorating rapidly. And although we tried to get hold of the next of kin, you, or other family members, the fact is her illness was progressing at such a rate that I do not think we would have reached an agreement with you before her heart stopped. And I do not wish for my patients to undergo resuscitation by default. Just because the treatment is theoretically available does not mean it should be given to every patient. That would be in unthinking way of practising medicine. And although you are right, it would have been ideal for her, and if not her then you, to have been involved, it is I who would have been responsible for any side effects from that treatment. And those side-effects are not minor. I don't really wish to describe them in detail to you now when you are grieving, but you undoubtedly know about them.

S: Yes of course. Cracked ribs…brain damage. We know all about those. But if there is a chance of life afterwards surely that outweighs all of those factors. Wouldn't you agree that the continuation of life is worth it? Don't you think so? Life!

C: We concern ourselves primarily with the quality of life rather than its duration.

S: I know you do. Quality over quantity. But surely that assessment requires more information about what the patient would want. Before deciding where they lie on that set of scales you must involve them, or if not then their family. Because your assessment of quality, is coloured by the many bad things that you have seen in medicine. You have a jaundiced view. You must not be allowcd to make unilateral decisions.

C: You have a point there. My experience of seeing patients who never recover from resuscitation, instead spending weeks in a intensive care unit, in a sedated state, or deteriorating in a ward, unable to feed themselves, may have coloured my view. But I don't think that makes me less qualified to make a decision...rather it makes me more qualified. That knowledge reinforced the sense of duty I feel...to protect patients from that fate... from that vision of recovery that I know converts into reality very rarely indeed. Life itself is precious, I agree, but a life allied to suffering, without meaningful communication with loved ones, is I would argue a life that is not worth living. I believe that.

S: So you are deciding whose lives are not worth living. That is what I suspected. It is completely unilateral. There is too much power in your hands. And I will not be so rude as to enter into other factors that might be influencing you. Such as worrying about how long such patients will remain in your hospital, using up intensive care facilities. Or the money that are spent on them. We won't go there...

C: I can assure you that those factors do not enter my mind. When I look after a patient like your mother my only thoughts are for their well-being. But we need to think about how she was before she died. We been talking about how she might have been after

159

resuscitation, and I feel that I cannot convince you that the small chance of a successful result was not sufficient to risk the suffering that resuscitation can cause. But let us imagine what she was like when she was alive. Do you mind? I don't mean to be insensitive.

S: Go ahead.

C: Have you seen a person die?

S: No.

C: I will describe it for you. It can happen gradually or suddenly. The person who was once talking can arrest and all discernible functions will cease. When this happens the chance of a successful result is perhaps greater because, sometimes, you can just as rapidly the heart back into a normal rhythm. But even then in a very frail patient shock to the system is too great for long-term recovery. But in your mother's case it was a more gradual process. She came in talking, eating, functioning albeit weakly, but the chest infection did not respond and soon she did not have energy to eat or drink, was unable to bring a cup to her lips. Her heart was still beating yes, but she turned her head to one side.

I can never tell what patients are thinking when they have reached the stage, or if they are forming thoughts at all. What I can say is that the life that they have is purely internal. There is no exchange of ideas with those around them, at most perhaps an indication of how they are feeling or perhaps a flicker of recognition. And you must bear in mind that this is how they are *before* the heart stops. So if you ask me why I did not try to resuscitate your mother I must make it clear that the level of existence that she had prior to her heart stopping was one that I feel sure she would not have wanted to return to. Can I say with certainty that she could not have been brought back to better state than that? Not 100%, of course…but I can be certain that that was the most likely outcome. She did not die without warning. We had seen the signs of deterioration, and knew that within hours, a couple of days at the very most, her heart would give out. She was already receiving the maximum amount of treatment that we could give. Her heart stopping was a natural end to her illness.

S: You say she was on as much treatment as you could give. You explain that her heart was already weakening. But what about intensive care?

C: Intensive care is not for all. It is not automatic if patients deteriorate. Intensive care, if offered indiscriminately, is sometimes a drawn-out attempt at resuscitation. And it brings with it the potential harms, such as invasive ventilation and sedation, that resuscitation would invoke within a few minutes. In intensive care those treatments are added sequentially as parts of the body fail. But it is because we know that recovery is so unlikely that we do not send all of our patients there.

S: So by saying that she would not appropriate for intensive care you are implicitly saying that she was not appropriate for resuscitation?

C: That is true.

S: You cannot have one without the other?

C: If the patient is not referable to intensive care, it is not reasonable to resuscitate. Because after resuscitation you know that they will need intensive care. You cannot have one without the other.

S: So why are these issues not explained upfront? Why when she came into hospital was it not explained that she would not go to intensive care?

C: It is like discussing a treatment that you know will never be relevant. It's like talking about chemotherapy if a patient does not have cancer.

S: I don't follow that. It's an irrelevant parallel.

C: I'm trying to illustrate that if a form of treatment has no place in a patient's treatment plan there is little point in talking about it. It confuses patients, leads them to consider options that do not exist.

S: But again you can't pretend to know people feel about the preservation of life. It does not seem relevant to you because you are comfortable that a patient like my mother should be allowed to die without resistance. But the families of your patients will not always agree. The families of your patients have lived with those individuals their whole lives. Their death is more than the end result of another presentation of severe pneumonia. Their death is the destruction of a library of memories and experiences. It cannot be accepted without more discussion and thought.

C: I understand your point. But that accumulation of experience and memories is not respected by disease. Pneumonia affects people without discrimination or favour. And we know that disease well. Whatever the individual circumstances or experiences of our patients, and whatever their relationships, the disease will do what it will do and the patient's organs will resist or succumb in complete ignorance of the value that the individual puts on their life. The backdrop that scenery of emotional parts will make no difference from a medical point of view. I do not wish to be cold or overly clinical, but that is the truth.

S: But it is that attitude – doctor – that leads us to accuse you of brutalisation. You portray the patient as a collection of organs fighting a disease. And that results in a shrinkage of respect for everything else that patients bring into hospital with them. That shrinkage makes you less inclined to do everything in your care to understand the patient in the context of their family life. You see

163

another severe case of pneumonia in an elderly person and you know, the moment you see that patient, or my mother, they will probably die. Only that does not cause you much distress because you have already seen ten in the last fortnight. It is inevitable...it is automatic, for you.

C: That is a very harsh accusation. You're accusing me of valuing the lives of our patients to a lesser extent then their families.

S: But doctor, be honest with yourself. That must be true. You do not love these patients. If one of them dies you will go home and carry on your life. So don't pretend that you value these lives as much as you value the lives of your own family. What I am asking you to consider is that you remind yourself how important those lives are to the families that you try, as you say – half-heartedly I say – to get hold of.

C: We do that. We are sensitive to these issues. You paint an unfair picture of us.

S: Then why only a single attempt to contact me? Why was a nurse not trying every avenue to get hold of me or one of the other family members. It would not have taken much effort or gumption. It was just not a priority for you, your team. You knew what was going to happen and that you could not stop it. I'm beginning to accept that, I respect your medical opinion. But why allow that to happen without doing everything in your power to bring us to the bedside earlier? I'll tell you why. Because death is routine for you. For all of you. Common, frequent, a daily occurrence, a column on the chart...routine! So for you, death does not bring with it the sense of crisis, a frisson of the exceptional, that it does for the families. This must be the explanation. Death is inevitable...you surrender to it – on behalf of your patients – and you move on...

C: We don't...

S: Have time? I don't care...

C: I wasn't...

S: You move on, to concentrate on those whom you may be able to save. It's important work, we accept that. You fight nature, march onwards across many battlefields, and cannot spare the time to stay behind with the dying or the dead, for nothing that you can do will save them. To do so would distract you, divert your valuable energies. I get that. But as the memories of the dead recede in your own mind, they enlarge and dominate the lives of the relatives. It is a crisis for them. Death, however it arrives, inevitable or no – and who am I, really, to argue with about that? – is a special moment. We need to be involved. Lack of involvement lends it an air of... insignificance, throwaway. We know that tomorrow another will die, and another, and another, but we don't care about that. We can only think about *our* death. That's where you, or the system you work in, fails. By not allowing space – physical, emotional, temporal - to develop around the deaths that you manage.

C: I...I can't defend the lack of privacy you experienced, I know that is not ideal, but regarding of your belief that we are not affected by death, and do not allow it to slow us down...I cannot agree with that. We do remain sensitive to death. We have relatives to, most of us will have experienced death in the family. We are not automatons.

S: Are you sure? In this hospital, rushing around, moving your patients through, are you sure that you permit yourself the luxury of *feeling* how important each death is?

C: Not to the same extent as the importance felt by the family, that would be unrealistic...

S: But enough...enough to put other things aside, and make each death, or even before death, the prospect of death, to make each one special? If you did, and if the members of your team did, they would have found me or one of my siblings, before you made the decision not to resuscitate. In this case doctor, my mother's case, the discrepancy between your team's perception of her death's significance, and ours, was huge. That's why we are here isn't it? You made a decision without us, and we believe that is not what she would have wanted. And you did not give yourself the opportunity to convince us otherwise. You thought it would be 'just fine'…because it's just so obviously right to you! Do you understand what I'm saying?

The End.

[The case is fictional]

A form of words: honesty kindness, coercion and early resuscitation discussions

As doctors are encouraged to address the issue of resuscitation at an ever earlier stage following admission to hospital, the problem of how to introduce the subject becomes more acute. If sufficient thought is not given to the challenge, there is a risk of coercion, especially in more elderly patients.

Studies and audits of patients who have undergone cardiopulmonary resuscitation (CPR) show that in many cases it would have been appropriate for a DNAR instruction to have been put in place before the cardiac arrest. To put it simply, the clinical information available made it clear that CPR was always going to be futile. Even if patients do not appear unstable it is sensible to discuss the risks and benefits of resuscitation with those who are frail and elderly. A large epidemiological study of patients in the U.S. who underwent CPR (William J. Ehlenbach et al, NEJM, 2009) found that 12.2% of those aged over 90 years survived to discharge. This result is at the optimistic end of the spectrum: other studies have found 0% survival in those over 90 years, and one found that for every survivor over 80 years of age, 29 would need to undergo resuscitation (David Paniagua et al, Cardiology, 2002).

One could argue that patients should consider whether they would like to be resuscitated or not even before they are admitted to hospital. There is certainly a drive now to encourage patients to think about end of life scenarios while they are stable, at home and completely clear in their thoughts (for instance the National End of Life Care Programme). Once they are admitted to hospital it is common for patients to lose the capacity to make fully informed decisions. It is at this time that doctors are required to canvas the opinion of the patients' loved ones and work out what they would have preferred and to make their medical decision within that context. As we know from cases that have recently been referred to the Court of Protection the wishes of the patient or their family are not always congruent with the medical team's opinion.

The ideal therefore is for patients to have engaged with this question before they become unwell. The next best thing is to engage them in the topic once they have been admitted to hospital, but before the worst happens. Indeed there is a growing expectation that resuscitation decisions (be they For... or Not for...) be made at the first consultant review following admission, and certainly within 48-72 hours (NCEPOD, Time To Intervene).

So how do we raise a subject in busy clinical environments or in situations where the last thing on the patient's mind is the possibility that their heart might stop?

Optimum approaches have been explored before. An article by Charles F von Gunten, published in the Journal of Clinical Oncology (2001), presented a 6 step model:

1. Establish an appropriate setting for the discussion.

2. Ask the patient and family what they understand.

3. Find out what they expect will happen.

4. Discuss a DNR order, including context.

5. Respond to emotions.

6. Establish and implement the plan

The sense of this algorithm cannot be doubted. The reservation I have is that a post-take round does not provide for the conditions that are required for it to work. There is little privacy, the relevant family members may not be present, and responding to the emotional fall-out can take up more time than is easily afforded in the pressure to see each patient.

For these reasons, and others, it is clearly unrealistic for consultants to address the question with every frail or very elderly patient, but nevertheless the proportion of patients to whom we have a responsibility to initiate this engagement is surely growing. It is not a callous trend; it has nothing to do avoiding active treatment – it is just an awareness that unless we bring the subject up there is a risk that our patients will be subjected to inappropriate, unpleasant measures *by default.*

To me it is about finding the right form of words. It is also about balancing gentleness and sensitivity with the stark reality that resuscitation rarely works in the very elderly, frail population.

This is how I do it. It is not meant to presented as an ideal, and I would welcome other examples if medical practitioners wish to reply on the blog.

So, imagine I am seeing a 92 year old lady who lives in her own home. She has moderate aortic stenosis and mild kidney disease. She had a minor heart attack in her eighties. She has a chest infection. At a push she might have been discharged on oral antibiotics from A&E, but it is 10 o'clock at night and that feels inappropriate. She has been breathless for a few days and needs some time in hospital. Most would agree, the chance of her arresting is low, but the chance of her being successfully resuscitated is even lower. Should I bring it up? Well, I do. After the history presentation from my SHO, a brief physical examination and perusal of the drug chart, I say,

"Mrs Evans, I'd like to discuss something with you. It may sound rather pessimistic and serious, but it is important that we talk about it. I need to ask you about what we should do if your heart were to suddenly stop. As you probably know, for some patients we try to restart the heart with compressions on the chest and electric shocks, but we do know that this does not work very well as you become more frail, or of you already have problems with the heart or the lungs.

"It's important that we understand your feelings about this, and write it in the notes so that other doctors can know what to do if something like that were to happen. But I must emphasise, that based on your results, the blood tests, heart tracings and the chest x-ray, I don't think there is a very high chance of this happening. But I like to ask all of my patients - as it is an important subject."

I have had many responses, across a broad spectrum:

Bewilderment:

"Oh...I've never really thought about that before doctor. I didn't think I was that unwell."

Defiance of mortality:

"Well I want to live as long as I can. I don't want to give up that easily."

Fatalism:

"Whatever happens, it's meant to be..."

The 'old fashioned', those who are comfortable with a thoroughly paternalistic style:

"Do whatever you think is best…"

The sure:

"No. no, I definitely wouldn't want that, I've had quite enough time."

And the hesitant,

"OK doctor, but I would like to discuss with my family. They would want to be involved."

The latter response presents a further challenge. The patient clearly has capacity to express their wishes. But, presented with this dramatic scenario of the heart stopping, they immediately refer to their loved ones. That is natural. Where else would you turn when suddenly confronted with an image of dying. Thus, another step has been introduced. It is vital that doctors do not proceed unilaterally, and only the foolhardy or unthinking would do so. But compliance with the patient's wishes, and all guidelines regarding end of life decisions, must be balanced by honesty; why was I asking that question? Because I knew what *I thought* the answer *should* be. I asked it because I did *not* think that resuscitation would be successful or the right thing to do. Therefore, my question was a loaded one, even though I approached it in a very open manner. Now my goal, that of 'achieving' a DNAR decision, has been postponed. How do I proceed?

I may push a little harder, acutely aware of the danger of coercion.

"Well, it's understandable that you would want to discuss it with your daughter, and I am certainly happy to wait for you to do that. But I do think it is important that you tell us what you think and that we tell you what we think. Again, I have to say that I'm only bringing this up because I don't want there to be any confusion should your heart suddenly stop. And although it hasn't given you much trouble recently it's only sensible for us to go into it. The trouble is that based on our experience there will be only a small chance that we could get your heart beating properly again, and there would be a possibility of damage to the brain or prolonged recovery on intensive care with mechanical ventilators etc. Have you thought about this sort of thing before, at home? Some people have seen friends who have needed life support machines…"

The patient still prefers to wait and discuss it with family members. What do I do?

In situations where there is no urgency, such as the scenario I have described here, I let it go. I will have done a good job in introducing the subject and bringing the family unit together to think about this important decision. That is a difficult word – *decision*. Although I have tried not to portray it as a simple 'yes' or 'no', there is now the danger that the family will meet on their own, without a member of the medical team to frame the discussion. The end result, and I have seen this, may be that the next of kin approaches a ward nurse later to say,

"The consultant asked my mother to discuss resuscitation when he saw her yesterday. She's has a good think, with us, and she has decided you should do it." Now, having appeared to transfer the onus of decision making to the family unit I have misled them. They believe that the decision is made, but in reality the outcome, 'for resuscitation' remains medically inappropriate – in my view.

The situation is more difficult when I feel that the patient is unstable and that a resuscitation decision would ideally be made before they leave the department, or at most within 12 hours of arrival in the medical assessment unit. In these circumstances waiting for the family to come in and for a full discussion to take place is difficult. Here the medical view begins to predominate…and it is here that we risk bulldozing patients into an assent.

If I have made up my mind that resuscitation is definitely inappropriate, and the patient remains ambivalent, there is a temptation for me to give more and more depressing detail about how poor this treatment is, who violent, how brutal, until they submit and say 'OK Doctor, I respect your opinion, I had no idea it was that bad… I don't want that to happen to me'. The end result is an appropriate decision, and an appropriate document will be placed in the notes. However, this approach risks later complaints from family members who feel differently, or more importantly know that that the patient feels differently. It is this combination of circumstances that has resulted in court appearances for doctors and their trusts.

So what do I advise now, in the case of an *unstable* but still capacitous patient? The patient remains ambivalent…but I am certain. Clearly the family need to be brought in. But there will be a time delay. I am committed elsewhere with other emergency patients. Do I risk being diverted away from this important decision so that it remains unresolved until the next working day? What if the patient does arrest. They will be resuscitated by default. They will probably die and I will feel guilty that I allowed inappropriate, uncomfortable and undignified treatment to proceed because I did not have the courage to fill out the document. I did not have the courage because I knew that I would be opening myself to criticism by the family if they had not been involved and disagreed.

So I call the family myself. I get through to the nominated next of kin, whose details are listed in the notes. I explain the need to further this discussion. It is a difficult situation because the patient has capacity and I am not asking for their 'substituted judgement'. But the patient is ambivalent and I do need assent. So am I asking family members to take the place of the patient? No – I am seeking consensus. And I am protecting myself from accusations of bullying and over persuasion.

The person I call may be just as ambivalent. They may be even less likely to have considered the question of end of life care as it relates to their parent, because they are younger. So what I am doing is forcing an accelerated emotional and intellectual engagement with a very difficult subject. It feels a little cruel. But I steel myself knowing that it is necessary and that if the end result is a peaceful death for a patient who would never recover from CPR then I have done a good thing.

Will I ever fill out a resuscitation form without waiting for a consensus? I will if I know that the patient is deteriorating and likely to die within hours. That is because the natural history of disease has revealed itself as irreversible and inexorable. Nature has revealing itself and death appears certain. In this situation resuscitation is irrelevant, and no doctor would allow it to happen.

In conclusion, I have attempted to portray the subtleties, challenges and risks of early resuscitation discussions. It would be a lot easier if individuals gave a thought to end of life care before they become patients, but it is easy to understand why the issue tends to come to a head only in the context of acute illness. Suffice to say, the difficult words that need saying after admission to hospital are chosen carefully, and however brutal they sound, the thought processes behind them are well intentioned.

177

Painful procedures at the end of life: a growing dilemma in healthcare for the elderly

My niece spent a week shadowing me for work experience recently. Most sessions were with helpful colleagues, but I brought her into one of my endoscopy sessions. I looked forward to showing her how interesting it was. In the car, on the way home at the end of the week, I asked her if she was still keen on medicine,

"Definitely. I loved the surgery..but I couldn't do what you do, I couldn't hurt people."

That got me thinking! The realisation that being a doctor involves inflicting pain is quite shocking and unpleasant for medical students. For me it came in the fifth year, when I started doing phlebotomy rounds every morning. Particular patients, listed for daily venesection, would wince as they caught sight of me entering their bay. After the third failed stab I had to pause and ask myself if it was reasonable to continue. But I did, only giving up after five attempts. The fact that each episode of pain represented a tiny step up the learning curve made me feel even more guilty. Now, as a consultant, I am not removed from the dilemma of 'therapeutic pain'.

§

Here is a scenario (the details have been changed from reality, as normal). A previously rather impressive, but moderately demented 91 year old lady is admitted with pneumonia. She had been living at home, assisted by carers who visit twice a day. The infection causes delirium, and despite some improvement with antibiotics it becomes clear that her strength and overall level of function have taken a significant hit. On the ward rounds and board rounds doctors, nurses, physiotherapists and occupational therapists begin to discuss the intensity of the care package that she will require. It is felt that the most realistic option will be a residential home.

She enters a period of stability and the doctors spend a little less time with her each day – there is very little to do, medically speaking.

One day she passes some altered, darkened blood on the toilet. Her blood count falls. It is supposed that she has bled from a gastric ulcer, and an endoscopy is arranged. Her family are informed, and a Consent Form 4 is completed. This is the type of consent form that doctors write on when a patient does not have the mental 'capacity' to make up their own mind if they actually want the procedure. In this case the doctors agree that the endoscopy, although unpleasant, is brief and straightforward enough to be justified, 'in her best interests.' She has the procedure, under the minimum dose of sedation…and no ulcer is found. The endoscopist writes 'procedure poorly tolerated' on the report. Next day she has no memory of having the camera passed through her mouth into her stomach.

She remains stable. Two days later she bleeds again, and is transfused another two units of blood. The team arrange a CT scan to look for a bowel tumour –it doesn't show one, but the radiologist suggests that the caecum (90cm into the bowel) is examined directly. They choose to wait again, reluctant to submit her to a colonoscopy.

She bleeds again. Another two units. Each episode of blood loss weakens her a little. The medical decision is, on the face of it, easy…she needs a colonoscopy. But this test is difficult for elderly patients. It requires that the bowel is cleaned thoroughly with strong laxatives, before the endoscope is negotiated through entire length of the large bowel. The elderly tend to have angulated, inflexible colons, factors that make the procedure more uncomfortable. It is no small thing to arrange such a test for a 91 year old.

Her family are informed of events again. Colonoscopy is explained in some detail. 'What will happen if she doesn't have it?' her son asks. She will bleed again, and require another transfusion. It could go on and on. She will not be able to leave the hospital. It is likely that she her health will deteriorate and she will succumb to a complication. The fact that there is limit to the amount of blood that can be given to patient is not discussed. 'Can you put her to sleep for it this time?' The answer is no. A general anaesthetic is out of the question in such a frail lady. The family agree that she should have the colonoscopy. After all, it is usually safe, and she managed the other one pretty well. It is arranged.

§

It was I who did the first endoscopy. It started well but after thirty seconds she became distressed and tried to pull the camera out. I asked a nurse to hold her hand while I finished the test. She fought and dug her nails into the nurses palm. I was relieved to hear that she couldn't remember a thing afterwards.

It was my list that she was booked onto for her colonoscopy. I didn't recognise the name when I arrived in the department and read my patient list, but when her turn came towards the end of the afternoon I went out to consent her, I sighed. She appeared frailer, and could barely engage me in conversation. Another Consent Form 4 had been filled out, and I duly countersigned it, thereby adding my weight to the decision that had been taken on her behalf.

I gave the sedation (as much as I could safely give) and started the procedure. Within minutes, as the camera began to stretch and twist the part of the bowel affected by diverticular disease (almost universal in the elderly), she began to object. I carried on, sure that within a couple of minutes the worst would be over for over. But it wasn't, and her cries became louder. I changed her position, I used every endoscopic trick, and a centimetre at a time progressed along the bowel. Facile words of encouragement from myself or the endoscopy nurses, such as 'You're doing very well,' 'Concentrate on your breathing…not too much longer now,' and 'You're completely safe, it's worth it to find out what's wrong…' did no good. She wasn't listening, and we had already determined that she was not able to process the information that was given to her. That's not to say she couldn't talk. As the procedure continued she began to say, then shout, with great clarity,

"Stop it!"

After the fourth or fifth 'Stop it' I stopped. Another five to ten minutes and I would have reached the caecum. I was already seeing signs of bleeding, trickling down the walls of the bowel from a lesion further in. I could get there, I had no doubt about it. I could make a diagnosis and perhaps even stop the leakage of blood. But it would mean at least five minute of pain, inflicted against her clearly expressed wishes.

What should I do? I asked the two nurses. They shrugged, uncomfortable with their patient's pain but experienced enough to know how important it was to find out what was causing the bleeding.

This was the question I had to ask myself. Did I think that it was better for the patient to suffer for as long as it took me to find the problem and seal the blood vessel, to be saved further transfusions, or achieve instant relief by removal of the camera, thus forfeiting the chance of a cure. It was up to me. Present pain (audible, visible, horrible to witness) versus future health (theoretically).

I carried on. I usually do. It had been discussed with the family. Her doctors had considered the pros and cons of the procedure in some depth. I explained this to the more doubtful and distressed of the two nurses, and together we got the frail old lady through it.

I found nothing. We never made a diagnosis.

I went to see her the next day, and introduced myself. She remembered nothing. Is amnesia the same as analgesia? I don't think so. She suffered in that endoscopy room, at my hands.

§

I explained some of these thoughts to my niece at a later date, but I didn't make much of an impression. The pain was very real for her too, and her opinion, as an 'innocent', unbiased by the utilitarian, task-oriented approach that doctors sometimes take, seemed very valid. Whatever the justification, we – the team, her relatives, me – judged that she would have wanted to trade pain for the chance of cure. The more I reflect on this equation, the more I doubt it's solution. As our patients become older and less able to give

184

informed consent we are going to have to address this issue in greater detail. Every disease has a treatment. We are used to analysing the ratio of discomfort to benefit for our patients, but the more I treat such 'very' elderly patients, the greater the weight I give to the present rather than future state of health with which we choose to justify pain.

A soft task hard to do: why we fail in engaging relatives at the end of life

Every controversial end-of-life decision that I have read about in recent months has had one thing in common: inadequate communication. They appear to have progressed to the courts or the newspapers because doctors made decisions without ensuring that families were in agreement. The most frustrating aspect of these widely publicised cases is the realisation that half an hour spent in a quiet room discussing the reasons, explaining the pros and the cons, might have halted the subsequent polarisation of views. The fact that the decision was being made to protect the patient, and not bring forward their death, could have been emphasised. The family's understanding of what their loved one's probable view on the subject could have been explored. An ambivalent or frankly negative response might have alerted the team to the fact that their patient's family had a concrete view on resuscitation or end of life care.* Having tested the temperature, the medical team could have stepped more tentatively into the ethical waters that were soon lapping over their beleaguered heads.

Here I explore some of the reasons why doctors sometimes fail in the task of engaging families in end of life discussions.

1) The pressure to make early decisions

In 2012 a report published by the National Confidential Enquiry into Patient Outcome and Death (NCEPOD) called 'Cardiac Arrest Procedures: Time To Intervene' showed that there are systematic weakness in our care of patients before and after cardiac arrest. They reviewed the notes of hundreds of patients who had arrested and undergone cardiopulmonary resuscitation. An important component of this poor performance was inadequate identification of frail patients who are not likely to survive resuscitation. Essentially, we are attempting to resuscitate too many patients. The investigators found that only 52 of 552 patients had a DNAR decision, but at least 196 should have based on the clinical information available. Potentially therefore, those without a DNAR decision were subjected to resuscitation attempts that were always going to have a very low chance of success.

Mr Bertie Leigh, Chair of NCEPOD, wrote in his foreword to the report:

'Alas, the results are profoundly disappointing and as I read these pages I wondered how many of these interventions would be defensible if charged as assaults before the criminal courts, or as professional misconduct before the GMC. The GMC recognises that CPR should be administered in an emergency, but it is not good medical practice to fail to anticipate the needs of the patient before an emergency arises. If the failure is deliberate or reckless

then I suggest that it is arguably criminal. In the overwhelming majority of cases the question of CPR was not raised with the patient before the arrest...'

The NCEPOD report has resulted in an increased awareness that delayed resuscitation decisions reflect bad organisation and bad practice within hospitals. The pressure is on, to make these decisions soon after admission, in the first 24 to 72 hours. The question is, are doctors equipped to broach end of life subjects at such an early stage? And are families going to be prepared for it?

2) *The nature of emergency*

Emergency medicine presents specific hurdles to good communication. Patients themselves are often too unwell to engage. Due to the unforeseen nature of their presentation, perhaps in the middle of the night or the early hours of the morning, the most important members of the family are frequently absent. Phone calls can be made, but if a patient is deteriorating quickly and the doctor's strong conviction is that resuscitation would be useless, a DNAR form will have to be completed – even without a discussion. Resuscitation decisions can usually wait until the next day of course, but even then it is challenging for doctors in this early period to arrange the necessary meetings. Visiting hours can be restrictive. Senior team members may be tied up elsewhere, in clinics or meetings... NCEPOD investigators were unsympathetic to this argument:

'Only a minority of patients in this group had a cardiac arrest within 12 hours of hospital admission and that most were in hospital for one or more days. Lack of time appears to be a poor reason not to have made decisions about CPR status in this group.'

So much for the pressure of time. It is a weak excuse. Arrangements can always be made if sufficient priority is given to a task. It is the question of priority that cuts to the heart of this problem. Why don't doctors perceive these conversations as important enough to reschedule other, more routine commitments?

3) The business of a ward round

The primary aim for any acute medical team on a ward round is to see each patient on their list, make a comprehensive, accurate assessment of their problems, and formulate a management plan. If they do not manage to see those patients in the allotted time they will have failed. Following this, they must effect the decisions generated by each of those assessments. These are physical tasks that have immediate, or very short term, visible consequences. A septic patient needs another blood culture. A feverish man with confusion requires a lumbar puncture. An abdomen that is full of fluid requires draining. A phone call to a GP, to obtain more background history. A referral to the neurosurgeons. These tasks are important – if they are omitted the junior doctor will be answerable and the senior doctor embarrassed. The patient will not have progressed, their symptoms will not have been relieved. Their length of stay will be extended.

The significance of a family conference may pale in comparison to such 'hard' tasks.

4) Medical simplicity, emotional complexity

In many cases the question of resuscitation is so obvious that, to put it crudely, the decision is a 'no-brainer' for the medical team. A quick perusal of the medical notes, combined with a glance at the patient from the end of the bed, may be enough to persuade the team that resuscitation would not only be medically ineffective, but unkind. When the clinical impression is so immediate and strong, the need to relay this information to the family may appear less important. Where is the controversy? The family will undoubtedly agree, it's a clear cut case, isn't it? Hasn't the patient been deteriorating for weeks at home, under their very gaze? Surely they won't require a detailed explanation…

The mistake here is the assumption that something so medically uncomplicated will be equally straightforward from an emotional point of view. This error reveals a lack of empathy – or what I call 'extended empathy', an emotional exercise that demands an appreciation not only of the patient's feelings, but of the family's too.

5) Coasting

The number and complexity of medical tasks that are generated during a ward round has been mentioned already. The focus of the medical team is to identify pathology and to reverse it. Those tasks require concentration and application. Details cannot be missed and omissions cannot be tolerated. Junior doctors must navigate their way through unfamiliar systems in large organisations to get things done. But if the battle for a patient's life appears to be lost, and death becomes inevitable, the level of concentration required diminishes.

I would argue that doctors drop into a lower gear when managing the dying. The pressure, to save life, is off. No harm can be done now (except perhaps an inappropriate resuscitation attempt). The intense focus on defeating disease fades, and it is possible that other, equally important but physically less tangible tasks, are sidelined. This is not to say that the needs of the patient or their family are ignored, just that in the never-ending pressure to identify and hold disease in its tracks, smoothing the way for a cart that has already slipped its harness and is rolling inexorably down the hill appears less critical.

6) Brutalisation

This word was used in a <u>well-known newspaper</u> to describe society's attitude to death in the elderly population.

191

'The Liverpool Killing Pathway is driven not just by crude economic calculation but by a wider brutalisation of our culture, at the heart of which lies the erosion of respect for the innate value of human life.'

I took this personally (which doctor wouldn't?) and immediately rejected the word. But the more I reflected on the reports of poor practice elsewhere, the more I began to fear that the accusation contained a kernel of truth. In 2007 I published a paper called 'The Absence of Sadness: Darker Reflections on the Patient-Physician Relationship' (unlocked, J Med Ethics) in which I described how exposure to death and suffering can result in a neutral emotional reaction to death. It is of course a cliché that doctors slowly become nonchalant to death, but it cannot be denied that in order to cope with the incessant stream of death that flows through their workplace they do develop ways of compartmentalising tragedy. Perhaps an inevitable consequence of this is a failure to appreciate how much time is required to explain each one, and how important it is involve those family members who are affected by it.

If death is no longer remarkable to a doctor it is not surprising that they cannot prioritise the need to communicate and explain its arrival to a patient's family. If it appears routine then their approach to the task of talking will be just that – routine.

It would seem impossible to the right thinking observer that doctors can develop such inhuman frigidity, but we must consider the possibility. But we must also sympathise with a tendency to become unfeeling in this way. This is because death *is indeed* routine. Patients come to hospital to die. It may not be the best place for them to do so but it is frequently their final destination. Even if death is expected, in say a nursing home, it is often too much to expect the family or General Practitioners to manage it. So ambulances are called and patients are admitted. Frequently the fact that they are dying is no surprise at all. Not to the doctors involved, not to the family.

This is not to say that a detailed and sensitive explanation as to what might happen on the wall is not required. But for the doctor who has been asked to assess a dying patient, and who quickly concludes that this is the natural end to their life, it is hard to conjure up instant feelings of sadness that might then transform into a recognition of the need to communicate. There may be no sense of urgency. Only if the doctor becomes aware that the family are on a completely different page, and have no idea how close to death the elderly relative is, will the need to engage them become of paramount importance.

So what haven't we covered…oh, that's right…the patients and families themselves! But this is where my analysis must end. I can make a stab at understanding how doctors feel and behave, but those on the other side of the curtain, well, that's an infinitely variable world. To understand how they will react to end of life conversations, and how open they might be such approaches, we need to take into account education, religion, grief and personality, and that is beyond the ambition of this essay.

* This is not to say the medical decision would have been *altered* or *reversed*, but in offering a more detailed explanation, or agreeing to revisit the subject after family had been given time to reflect, the clash of opposing views might have been softened.

Note:

Recent controversial DNAR cases include those at <u>Addenbrookes</u> and <u>Queen Elizabeth the Queen Mother, Margate</u>.

Missed opportunities: the diagnosis of dying and the risks of delay

Controversy over the Liverpool Care Pathway (LCP) has crystallised the issues of prognostic accuracy, futility and treatment burden at the end of life.

The Telegraph, on the 29th October 2012, summarised <u>current areas of concern</u>, which included:

- that it is impossible for medical staff to predict when death is imminent – so the decision to start the LCP is at best guesswork and at worst a form of euthanasia imposed without consent

- *that by removing all drips, especially fluids, the diagnosis of death becomes self-fulfilling*

It is suggested that premature introduction of the LCP, before all therapeutic avenues have been explored or given sufficient time to work, leads to avoidable deaths. Some say the LCP should only be introduced once a fatal outcome has become absolutely certain. Moreover, because there is no infallible way of diagnosing impending death, it might be safer not to use it at all, but to let death arrive in its own manner while we continue to treat actively in the hope of achieving a cure. In that way palliation – the cessation of antibiotics or other futile therapies, the withdrawal of artificially administered fluids and food, and the use of sedating or painkilling drugs, cannot be said to have eradicated the chance, however small, of survival.

Diagnosing Death

The diagnosis of dying is certainly unscientific. Estimating the duration of its approach, coping with its capricious tendency to retreat and re-group before a final advance, talking the patient or their relatives through this period, are huge challenges. There are some generally accepted signs of impending death, and critics of the LCP would have us wait for these to develop before converting to a palliative paradigm. Such signs include labile pulse rate and blood pressure, hypothermia and poor temperature regulation, sweating, pallor, cyanosis, irregular breathing patterns, audible airway secretions and confusion. These are the signs of dying, certainly, but I would suggest that they are not a useful guide. By the time they develop we may have missed the chance of providing comfort and avoiding harm.

The challenge we face is not in recognising death as it happens, but in knowing at an early stage whom death has marked out. It is these patients who are at risk of receiving prolonged and aggressive treatment that will prove ultimately futile. The suffering that elderly patients experience as a result of their treatment is the 'burden' that doctors have become so concerned about. Significant pain, inadvertent injury, or even low level 'run of the mill' discomfort and indignity are difficult to justify if the end result is certain death.

It is this 'pre-pre-terminal' phase that demands our attention. We cannot afford to make mistakes in its identification, for the stakes (avoidable death) are too high. Patients who were put on the LCP before the signs of dying had become manifest, only to improve and survive, those who 'defied' their doctors, proved to sceptics that the LCP may be a lethal tool. These cases (link to examples 1 2 3) helped ignite the current furore. Because no doctor is *always* right, it is quite possible that nervous clinicians will now delay the LCP until the signs of death are irrefutable, unwilling to rely on their clinical experience. The result may well be more treatment, for longer. The overall burden of futile treatment may rise.

Withdrawing active treatment vs failure to escalate

Critics of the LCP are uneasy that active treatment can be withdrawn before the signs of dying have revealed themselves. Honesty is needed here. In many cases a decision will already have been made not to 'escalate' treatment even if improvement does not occur with first line therapies. An example would be limiting therapy for pneumonia in a very elderly patient to antibiotics and oxygen via a face mask but not transferring them to intensive care for mechanical ventilation; or attempting to kick start failed kidneys in a 90 year old with fluids, but not offering the life-saving option of dialysis. If basic therapies prove ineffective and it is decided to convert to a palliative approach, the withdrawal of those failed first line treatments (e.g. antibiotics and fluids) is no worse, in my view, than *not* escalating. So, while criticising the removal of an IV cannula or nasogastric feeding tube (visible actions, commissions), it must be borne in mind that more effective interventions may well have been withheld (invisible omissions). The essential point is that treatment has failed and its continuation will make *no difference* to the chance of survival. Only measures that increase or preserve comfort can be justified.

Could this failure of escalation be a conspiracy to under-treat? One might portray it that way. But if we did not set such limits every single patient would pass through intensive care before being allowed to die. They do not, because we have made a calculation, that the burden of such super-aggressive therapy is disproportionate to the chance of success. There is no generally accepted metric, no reproducible equation with which to benchmark these decisions. Each calculation is made using unique data – medical history, comorbidities, functional 'reserve'…and of course what is known or can be ascertained about the patient's preferences. At the end of the day it comes down to medical experience, lessons learnt from seeing hundreds of patients go through similar experiences.

We must be honest too, in admitting that there are questions of resource to be taken into account here. A society that makes almost infinite demands on its health service must agree where to draw the line…and offering hi-tech, complex and prolonged organ support to those with multiple co-morbidities, or those who are near the end of their natural life, is one of them.

Saving lives – our primary aim

The LCP debate has unfortunately focused the public's attention on many negative aspects of medical care: treatment failure, futility, decisions on who not to treat, treatment withdrawal. It should be emphasised that doctors devote more of their time to treating than not treating, and are always looking for opportunities to save life. We are optimists, and are more likely to over-treat than under-treat, with a tendency to increase the burden of treatment in the hope that a patient will gradually show signs of improvement than make a hasty decision to withdraw. But we cannot escape the fact that with an ageing, comorbid population we will do a disservice to many patients if we treat indiscriminately. It is a poor doctor who sees only the disease and not the whole patient, who uses every therapy, technology and resource even as patients continue to deteriorate, and who 'flogs' a failing, weakening body with no thought for the pain or discomfort that is being endured.

Substituted judgment and resuscitation: a case

A 65 year old patient with advanced airways disease is treated with non-invasive ventilation but ICU decide that full mechanical ventilation via an endotracheal tube is not justified. The junior doctor on call discusses DNAR with her, but she indicates that she would like to be resuscitated. In the morning I am called to the ward where her husband and family await. He saw her survive a similar illness three years ago, including prolonged ventilation via a tracheostomy. After discharge he retired early from his job to focus on her convalescence, and is proud that the care that he and the community team have provided saw her exercise tolerance improve from just a few yards on discharge to 100 yards. She remains significantly debilitated.

I discuss her condition, and raise the question of resuscitation. In his mind there is no question – she must be resuscitated. I explain that her very poor baseline lung function, and the severity of her current infection, mean that attempts to restart the heart are almost certain not to work. I do not mention that prolonged ventilation in ICU has been vetoed already. He insists, and refers to doctors who said the same last time, only to be proven wrong. But this is different, I explain, she is weaker. He will not assent. It is not appropriate to go on and on, and I leave him so that he can back to her. I cannot fill out the DNAR in the face of such emphatic disagreement, but I know that for the patient it is right. I suggest that we speak again in the afternoon, and that if there are signs of deterioration I will have no choice but to make her DNAR. I reflect that even if he makes a formal complaint, I must do what I think is right for the patient.

We talk again. He emphasises that she would want to be resuscitated. But she has worsened, and I sign the DNAR. I discuss it with colleagues, and the concept of the 'short code', or limited resuscitation, or, in my view, a fake attempt, is raised. I find that option inappropriate, on the basis that it is motivated by concern for the relative and the doctor, but cannot be interpreted as being in the patient's interest.

The patient deteriorates further, and I sit with the husband again, for the last time that day. He begins to see the truth of the situation, and no longer objects to the DNAR order. The patient dies relatively peacefully next day. So what does this anecdote demonstrate?

A DNAR decision was proposed, but the patient's closest relative, the one who would know her true preferences best, objected to this. He knew that she would have wanted to be resuscitated, having come this far, having proved doctors wrong before. But I remained steadfast, and spent a lot of time talking him through my reasons. In the face of ongoing deterioration he finally removed his objection. I knew that there was a risk that he would make a formal complaint, and this caused me considerable discomfort. But circumstances, and my unwavering position, in the end persuaded him. Autonomy, and substituted judgement, were overruled.

The truth is, resuscitation is a treatment, and no doctor will provide a treatment unless it has a good chance of working. The challenge we have, as healthcare professionals, is that of communicating how ineffective that treatment is likely to be in so many cases.

Part 7: Quick, topical medical ethics overviews

Futility redux, and reset

The futility debate has had its day, hasn't it? At its height between during the 1980's and late 1990's there were hundreds of publications on the subject, but a NEJM 'sounding board' article by Helft et al, 'The rise and fall of the futility movement' appeared to bring it to a natural end. The authors explored definitions, data, the importance of patients' autonomy versus physicians' autonomy, and attempts to resolve disputes. They described how there had been,

...an attempt to convince society that physicians could use their clinical judgment or epidemiologic skills to determine whether a particular treatment would be futile in a particular clinical situation.

In their conclusion, where the authors sought to explain why interest in the idea of futility had dwindled, they pointed out that the medical community,

...could not agree on underlying principles...there was no consensus on a specific definition of futility or on an empirical basis for deciding that further care would be futile. Those who

argued that the critical issue was autonomy could not agree on whether patients or physicians should have the final say.

Doctor-centric exercises in calculation appeared at odds with the need to take into account the views of patients or their representatives. The right decision always depends on communication and a mutual understanding of burdens and benefits, so purely objective estimates of futility appeared bound to fail. The paper ends with,

The judgment that further treatment would be futile is not a conclusion – a signal that care should cease; instead, it should initiate the difficult task of discussing the situation with the patient...Talking to patients and their families should remain the focus of our efforts.

That does not sound alien to anyone who practises in a patient-centred way. Nevertheless, futility is a word that continues to be used in every hospital, every day of the week. It remains relevant because no doctor wants to advocate treatment that is useless. Futility remains important. Yet, in the absence of definitions we continue to make qualitative assessments.

In the rest of this article I would like to explore what factors influence doctors' perception of futility?

Changing the guard

An intensive care consultant once explained to me that frequent rotations with his colleagues through the unit minimized the risk not only of fatigue, but of 'therapeutic boredom'. He meant that after a week of trying to improve patients who were barely able to stand still, he began to run out of ideas. He grew weary of the grinding, entropic drift towards death that no amount of physiological tinkering or pharmacological manipulation could reverse. The only remaining option, to withdraw, grew more and more reasonable. But come Monday a new consultant with a fresh pair of eyes and, perhaps, a new idea, might change tactics and bring about some improvement. It struck me that in this environment, a rarefied and unusual one I admit, a physician's personal definition of futility was hugely significant. But for the patient it was a definition that could change overnight. Surely, I reflected, matters of life and death should not be altered by the psychological state of the doctor in charge. But of course, they do.

The language of futility

Apparently small chances of survival can be interpreted in different ways, according to whether the doctor or the patient/family have a positive or negative overall 'feeling'. That feeling may be determined by previous experience with a patient. Here I imagine two scenarios* with an estimated 5% survival probability. In **scenario A** the brother of a socially isolated, middle aged woman with decompensated cirrhosis feels strongly that organ support should *not* be continued, in contrast to the view of

207

her doctors who feel there are reversible factors worth treating aggressively. In **scenario B** a man with cirrhosis who has deteriorated several times before is once again admitted to ICU. The doctor feels that ongoing support is not justified, but his son demands that they do *not* give up. The 5% number is invoked, although there is of course no way that the accuracy of this can be proven. It is quite common for such numbers to be brought up as an easily understood 'handle' by which families can grasp the situation. It's something I tend to avoid nowadays.

Scenario A

The female patient's (pessimistic) brother: Isn't it all futile? Five per cent your colleague said, when she was admitted. One in twenty. It's not a figure to put much hope in, is it? "Fifty-fifty" would sound bad enough.

Doctor: I suspect my colleague wished to impress on you how very ill she was, not to rob you of all hope. But she has survived the first 48 hours. The next few days will be crucial in telling us if she can get through this, depending on how her heart, lungs and kidneys respond.

Brother: And if she shows no signs of improvement, what will you do? Turn off the machines?

Doctor: We may limit the amount of life support and submit to the natural process. The nurses would know that she was dying, and would not call for doctors to give electric shocks or more drugs if her heart slows down and stops. It would be as peaceful as possible. But should we see positive changes, we must give her as much support as she needs, so that those improvements can be built on.

Brother: What positive changes? Less of the blood pressure drug, less oxygen? In my mind those changes would mean very little; she would still be needing the ventilator, she would still be on life support, covered in wires, knocked out, totally dependent. But you will detect signs of improvement, and the process will go on and on.

Doctor: It would not go on indefinitely. She, her body, will tell us if indeed the time has come to die, and we will not strive to reverse the inevitable.   ·

Brother: But isn't it obvious already? Do you *really* believe she has a chance…or are you saying these things because you are trained to be positive, to treat, treat, treat? You take her 5 per cent chance and channel all your efforts into it, all the heroic potential of modern medicine. For a child, for a 30, 40-year-old struck down by a heart at- tack, meningitis, leukaemia, yes, but for my sister, so weak, ruined by her addiction … it doesn't seem right.

Scenario B

The 'end stage' patient' s son: But your colleague spoke of a 5 per cent chance, 1 in 20. So his illness *can* be reversed, one in every 20 cases. It seems a good enough chance to try for. Or was your colleague being optimistic?

Doctor: I always try to avoid quoting numbers, they don't mean much in individual cases. I'm not saying that some recovery from this infection is impossible, but even if the other organs begin to function his liver will have deteriorated further in the meantime. He will remain on the ward, permanently confused I should think, just as he has been since his last infection...

Son: He recognized us on the ward. He smiled when he heard my voice.

Doctor: That's good, but please understand me, I'm describing what he *might* be, should he have the energy and luck to grab that 5 per cent chance. But I do not think he will be able to take that chance.

Son: But surely you are trained, if not obliged, to concentrate on that small percentage. If you can get him through this ... and if he remains stable on the ward, he can go on the transplant list again, get a new liver, and live another 5, 10, 15 years. The alternative is so good, shouldn't you try your hardest to make it happen?

We see the same statistic presented in two ways; for the female patient with the pessimistic brother 5% is worth fighting for...yet the same doctor tries to convince the male patient's son that he is concentrating too fixedly on that '1 in 20' chance. Ultimately, the doctor devalues the statistic entirely by resorting to a deterministic outlook – ' ..five out of 100 people in his situation might survive, but for him, as an individual, fate may already be decided'. Interpretation is physician dependent.

Divorcing statistics from individuals

As scientists we are trained to read papers and absorb numerical evidence, but, strangely, there is also a duty to disregard data as we approach individual patients. The mystery of numbers when applied to medicine is one on which a statistician can shed more light that me. In 'Where is the Individual in Statistics?', Linda Tickle-Degnen dwells on standard deviations and how to discern individual variability in large analyses. Fascinatingly, she quotes Stephen J Gould (the famous paleantologist and science communicator) who was diagnosed with abdominal mesothelioma in 1982:

'I am not a measure of central tendency, either mean or median. I am one single human being with mesothelioma, and I want a best assessment of my own chances—for I have personal decisions to make, and my business cannot be dictated by abstract averages. I need to place myself in the most probable region of the variation based upon particulars of my own case; I must not simply assume that my personal fate will correspond to some measure of central tendency.'

In 2003 <u>Gawain Shelford, a doctor, wrote about his own relationship with statistics (BMJ – £)</u> after being diagnosed with rectal cancer at the age of 39. He wrote in bold italics,

'The information that I want is not that 1 in 10 patients will benefit, but whether I am that one...'

and asked if we,

'haven't all been bamboozled into believing that statistics and evidence are really relevant in our care of the individual patient. We repeatedly advise patients as to the best treatments for their illness, or for preventing illness, without pointing out that we have no true idea as to whether the treatment will in fact benefit them as an individual.'

Experience and nihilism

So, statistics shouldn't necessarily drive day to day medical decision making. That's easy to absorb....they derive from large studies that appear abstract and meaningless outside our personal experience. But we are still busy compiling a personal database, one which will hold great power over us. Those who work with critically ill patients month after month, year after year, are bound to review (consciously or subconsciously) their own accumulated experience. We learn the lessons of our past efforts, and believe the results of those often rather qualitative calculations more than those that those they read about in papers. Such a personal approach was condoned by Lawrence Schniederman et al in their 1990 Annals of Internal Medicine paper, '<u>Medical futility: it's meaning and ethical implications</u>',

...we propose that when physicians conclude (either through personal experience, experiences shared with colleagues, or consideration of reported empiric data) that in the last 100 cases, a medical treatment has been useless, they should regard that treatment as futile.

But does such a steady accumulation of face-to-face encounters risk the development of bias? Perhaps an extended, bad run will skew the tone and result in a jaded view. The world-weary attitude we sometimes see in more senior doctors may reflect a career's worth of exposure to poor results in certain conditions. Where once they threw everything at particular patients in the hope that through modern medical techniques and drugs they could drag their patients into the small percentage who *might* do well, later on they submit to the inevitable. They pick their therapeutic battles in a highly selective way. In doing so they would contend that they protect patients and their families from false hope, needless interventions, pain that is divorced from the reward of a longer life...from futility. But we must beware the self-fulfilling prophecy. If, despite a history of failure, there remains a real, albeit small chance of survival, taking a conservative approach may actually *guarantee* that the chance is zero.

Optics and caring

The continuation of manifestly futile treatment was described in a New York Times article in 2010. A dying 2 year old with severe congenital abnormalities underwent a resuscitation attempt, apparently for the benefit of his or her parents. The physician's approach to futility was criticized because it seemed that his duty of care had transferred to the parents, who left the hospital 'with a feeling of wholeness'. Neonatology and paediatrics are very special in terms of the way the family unit is managed, but in adult medicine there are parallels to this case...where appearances become the focus, even after futility criteria have been met.

Imagine a young man who has hitherto been doing well during his treatment for, say, leukaemia – potentially curable. He develops a severe infection with associated multiple organ failure following a course of chemotherapy. Organ support is continued well beyond the point at which the medical team have accepted, internally perhaps, the survival is impossible. But it is accepted that treatment will continue until his heart stops – why? The detailed logistics of how organ support technologies are withdrawn requires great skill and sensitivity. Treatment that is quite futile may be carried on until family members have arrived to say their final farewells. And on some occasions, in our imagined scenario for instance, I wonder if the decision not to actively withdraw is less a symbol designed to comfort the family, more the fulfilment of a promise to the man himself. To maintain a commitment not to 'give up'. He and his team made a pact at the outset, to go through thick and thin. There may be a stage in treatment therefore, where the chances of success have dwindled to well within the margin of futility, but in circumstances where it has been understood that it will be *the patient* who gives the final signal for release (by dying, by the heart actually stopping) rather than the physician. The decision, to withdraw, is never made. The doctor allows futile to continue, confident that it is not causing harm, but knowing that it can do no good.

No wonder the medical community never agreed on the criteria for futility. But as Löfmark and Nilstun proposed in their Journal of Medical Ethics review 'Conditions and consequences of medical futility—from a literature review to a clinical model',

'the following two questions should always be separated in the clinical setting: "What may be regarded as a futile measure?" and "What is justified in futility situations?"

The question is not what is futile, but how to deal with that futility.

Reset

This exploration of the subject of futility has made me pause. I'm sure most doctors would admit to developing nihilistic tendencies is some areas. Areas in which we have less knowledge perhaps, areas in which we have less interest. Perhaps, now and again, it is necessary to step back, clear our minds of the vivid, negative examples from our recent past, overlook the statistics that cannot be applied to the individual, remind ourselves that the patient's prognosis should not depend on our state of mind...and reset.

* I used these dialogues in a 2008 paper called'Sophistry and circumstance at the end of life' (Communication and Medicine)

Quality of life projections: do doctors have any idea?

It might seem reasonable that doctors, who find themselves suddenly inserted into the midst of a patient's life, make quality of life (QoL) assessments. They communicate with patients and family members, discover all that there is to know about their background, their habits, vices and hopes, and form an opinion about how the disease will affect the future. But doctors are wary about quoting those opinions in documentation that pertains to ceilings of treatment or resuscitation. They know that if a decision is made on the basis of a 'poor QoL' and the patient or family disagree, the potential for criticism is huge. Accusations of arrogance, of pretence to omniscience, of a God complex, may follow.

Doctors make predictions about how things will turn out. That is an essential medical skill. We know that if the disease does not respond the patient will at best be weakened, and at worst will die. When the impairment results in inability to look after oneself, engage in conversation or interact with the world, in depression or in chronic discomfort, we begin to regard QoL as diminished. However, the very word 'diminished' suggests some sort of *measure* of quality. If a patient's QoL is said to be worse, it suggests that we have some sort of comparator. What is that comparator? Is it based on *our* definition. If so, that definition will be the product of *our* upbringing, culture, faith and life experience. By making comparisons between enjoyable lives and intolerably burdensome lives we allow our own values to influence the therapeutic process. Disentangling those subjective impressions from the actual experience of our patients is a huge challenge. Louise Aronson, a Geriatrician at the University of California, explored this issue in a New York times article recently ('Weighing the end of life'), and made the point,

'To many people's surprise, most of my patients are as satisfied with their lives as they were when they were less debilitated.'

So, for my own sake and others', I have looked into where we stand on the question of quality.

The case of David James

QoL issues were crystallised, dramatically, by a recent judgment in the Court of Protection concerning David James, a 67 year old man in a 'minimally conscious state' who could not leave intensive care. A hospital Trust applied for permission not to provide further organ support or resuscitation should he suffer another crisis, but the judge upheld the family's challenge. Although the Trust won an appeal, shortly before Mr James's death (on 31st January 2012), the first judgment is worthy of a detailed analysis.

An intensive care doctor, when asked about the appropriateness of continued organ support, explored (among other considerations) the patient's quality of life.

'In the highly unlikely event that DJ survives his current illness, he will not be able to function as the musician he was previously due to the neurological deficits (hemiparesis) that he has developed. I have collected significant evidence that leaves me with the view that DJ would prefer to be dead rather than be unable to make music.'

According to the judgment however,

'the only basis for this last observation was a conversation with a nursing sister who says that DJ had apparently told another member of staff early in his admission to intensive care that he would prefer to die than not be able to play the guitar. Not surprisingly, DJ's family has been distressed at the use to which Dr _ put this snippet of information. In his second report and in his oral evidence he retracted without further comment the observation about making music.'

Here we see how narrow insights into a patient's personal, non-medical, circumstances can buckle under the weight of the medical decisions that rest on them.

In the judgment, descriptions of DJ's interactions are given, and the difference in interpretation by medical staff and family members become clear.

For instance, the intensive care doctor provided this record of a family visit:

'MJ and PJ (relatives) arrived by the bedside; DJ showed clear signs of recognition, smiled at their approach and mouthed what appeared to be words. He seemed to know appropriately when asked if he was feeling alright by his wife. She combed DJ's hair, during which DJ smiled. DJ was given a paper to read by his son. DJ turned the pages with his left arm. It is not clear to me whether he was reading any of the articles or looking at the pictures in the paper, however he smiled while looking at the paper. During this time he put on and took off his glasses ... PJ encouraged his father to play a simulated keyboard on [an] iPad. DJ was clearly interested in the iPad and its mount. He could not play any recognisable tunes on the simulated keyboard, even after his son demonstrated several simple melodies. PJ then opened a communication program with pictographic representations of moods (for example: happy face/sad face/angry face) with a

written description under each picture. PJ asked his father to show him what emotion he was feeling. I did not see a consistent response from DJ. DJ appeared to enjoy watching videos on his son's phone.'

To me, a non-neurologist with no specific expertise in severe brain injury, the term minimally conscious seems a little harsh for this situation. Indeed the judge made this comment,

> *'...there is a spectrum of minimal consciousness extending from patients who are only just above the vegetative state to those who are bordering on full consciousness. I would add that to that extent the word "minimal" in the diagnostic label may mislead. I accept that he qualifies for a diagnosis of being in a minimally conscious state, but his current level of awareness when he is not in a medical crisis might more accurately be described very limited rather than minimal.'*

Another doctor invoked quality of life when justifying his view there should be no escalation in care if DJ suffer another episode of severe sepsis.

> *' I would argue that further treatment for septic shock with hypotension and any artificial renal support would not be of overall benefit to DJ as such treatments would not return him to his former pleasures in life. '*

And again, concerning the question of CPR...

'... the very real risk of lack of oxygen to the brain as a result of any protracted attempt would surely not be in DJ's best interest given his interest in life.'

His diminished ability to enjoy 'interest in life' is invoked as a reason not to resuscitate. The judge then writes of the doctor,

'He (the doctor) would not revise his opinion unless matters have improved to the point where DJ was interacting with staff and actively participating in physiotherapy.'

In contrast, family members provided evidence to show that he *was* interacting:

'JJ is DJ's daughter... She produced photographs showing him interacting with members of the family. She said that at the moment, he is not looking so unwell. He has put on some weight and looks more lively and alert. He cannot speak because of the tracheostomy but his face is expressive and the family is sure that he can lip-read questions such as "why aren't you in work?" or "are you going out tonight?" She says that he worries about them. He is interested in family events, news, music and the radio. He is interacting more with the iPad.'

And so to the judgment. 'General considerations' for and against further organ support are listed:

For:

Life itself is of value and treatment may lengthen DJ's life/He currently has a measurable quality of life from which he gains pleasure. Although his condition fluctuates, there have been improvements as well as deteriorations/It is likely that DJ would want treatment up to the point where it became hopeless/His family strongly believes that this point has not been reached/It would not be right for DJ to die against a background of bitterness and grievance

Against:

The unchallenged diagnosis is that DJ has sustained severe physical and neurological damage and the prognosis is gloomy, to the extent that it is regarded as highly unlikely that he will achieve independence again; his current treatment is invasive and every setback places him at a further disadvantage/the treatment may not work/the treatment would be extremely burdensome to endure/it is not in his interests to face a prolonged, excruciating and undignified death

The judge goes on to explore the process of 'best interests' assessments.

> '...the assessment of best interests of course encompasses factors of all kinds, and not medical factors alone, and reaches into areas where doctors are not experts...'

Finally, in deciding in favour of the family, he writes:

> 'Although DJ's condition is in many respects grim, I am not persuaded that treatment would be futile or overly burdensome, or that there is no prospect of recovery.
>
> In DJ's case, the treatments in question cannot be said to be futile, based upon the evidence of their effect so far.
>
> Nor can they be said to be futile in the sense that they could only return DJ to a quality of life that is not worth living.
>
> Although the burdens of treatment are very great indeed, they have to be weighed against the benefits of a continued existence.
>
> Nor can it be said that there is no prospect of recovery: recovery does not mean a return to full health, but the resumption of a quality of life that DJ would regard as worthwhile. The

references, noted above, to a cure or a return to the former pleasures of life set the standard unduly high.

I consider that the (medical) argument ... significantly undervalues the non-medical aspects of DJ's situation at this time.

Moreover, as Hedley J put it in NHS Trust v Baby X [2012] EWHC 2188 (Fam), a life from which others may recoil can yet be precious. ... In this case, DJ's family life is of the closest and most meaningful kind and carries great weight in my assessment.'

Being a doctor, one who naturally tends to side with other doctors in such arguments, I have re-read the last paragraph many times. It says it all. We, doctors, are poorly qualified as observers when it comes to making quality of life assessments. The information that we have is sparse, our insights into the satisfaction that can be gained from small things (fleeting familial interactions for instance) are tainted by bias, and the weight that we give to other factors, such as technical futility or even resource limitations are not relevant to the patient.

Fallibility of QoL assessments: the evidence

Every study on quality of life assessment that I have read comes up with the same conclusion – doctors do not do it well. For example, <u>Sleven et al</u> gave QoL questionnaires to 108 patients and their doctors. A four point scale (**FPS** – from 'very good' through to 'very bad') and a linear analogue self-assessment (**LASA**) scale for QoL, anxiety and depression was employed were used. The correlations between patients and doctors were poor, with most values between 0.3 to 0.4, where 1.0 equals a perfect match. The authors concluded,

'Firstly it is clear that doctors could not adequately measure QoL.' and, 'QoL is a concept that includes many subjective elements, and it is therefore perhaps not surprising that a doctor may not have the necessary knowledge of the patient's feelings to evaluate their QoL accurately'.

Another study, by <u>Perron et al</u>, analysed the assessments of cognitive ability, independence with activities of daily living, depression, social isolation and general QoL in 255 DNACPR patients, as made by 9 physicians. The results showed that,

'Physicians systematically underestimated their DNR patients' mental state and physical condition: 23.9% of patients with a normal MMSE were considered by their physicians to be mentally abnormal, 28.7% with a normal ADL score were seen as physically moderately or totally dependent. Forquality of life, they misclassified 44.1% of the patients reporting a good quality of life.

'

They concluded,

'Our two main results were, first, that quality of life intervenes in more than 70% of the DNR decisions taken by the medical staff. Thus, when implementing a DNR order, physicians are very often influenced by their perception of patients' quality of life. Second, physicians systematically underrate their DNR patients' quality of life components (including mental state, physical and social condition, degree of pain and depression).

and,

'These discrepancies may be attributable to working in an acute care setting, where the physician-patient relationship is superficial and centred on diagnosis and treatment.'

Other studies show that we may have the wrong idea about long term outcome after resuscitation. De Vos et al found that of *'827 resuscitated patients, 12% (n = 101) survived to follow-up.'* This appears to confirm what we know, that CPR is not in itself a particularly effective treatment. However,

'Most survivors were independent in daily life (75%), 17% were cognitively impaired, and 16% had depressive symptoms. Factors during and after resuscitation, such as prolonged cardiac

227

arrest and coma, did not significantly determine the quality of life or cognitive functioning of survivors. The quality of life of our CPR survivors was worse compared with a reference group of elderly individuals, but better than that of a reference group of patients with stroke.'

...and this leads to the conclusion that,

'Cardiopulmonary resuscitation is frequently unsuccessful, but if survival is achieved, a relatively good quality of life can be expected. '

i.e.: if you survive you may do quite well. So is it necessary for us to agonise quite so much over QoL in the context of resuscitation? If the patient dies they will not suffer a poor QoL (only the indignity of the CPR attempt), but if they survive, the generally accepted wisdom that their existence will be blighted by bodily disability, dependency on others and depression, may not be true.

It is still necessary for us to consider who may or not survive of course, and the de Vos study did find that two factors were independently associated with poor outcome – the 'reason for admission' and 'age'. Although age does matter, we do not use chronological age when documenting DNACPR decisions. Of itself it is over-simplistic and does not take into account the great variation in underlying fitness that exists. However, at the upper extreme of human life expectancy, it is perhaps forgivable, as long as sufficient weight is given to underlying health issues and pre-existing organ dysfunction.

Current guidance

The Resuscitation Council gives the following advice, in situations where the burden of treatment appears to outweigh the benefits (i.e. poor projected QoL).

'These difficult situations are a potential source of confusion. Doctors cannot be required to give treatment contrary to their clinical judgement, but should be willing to consider and discuss patients' wishes to receive treatment, even if it offers only a very small chance of success or benefit. Where attempted CPR has a reasonable chance of successfully re-starting the heart and breathing for a sustained period, and patients have decided that the quality of life that can reasonably be expected is acceptable to them, their wish for CPR should be respected'

Here then, greater weight is given to the patient's understanding of quality than to the doctor's. In the rare cases where the doctor feels unable to agree with this, such is their conviction that CPR is wrong, obtaining a second opinion or a legal decision is suggested.

And what of the GMC? Its guidance 'End of life care: Discussion about whether to attempt CPR' includes this paragraph:

132. ... You must approach discussions sensitively and bear in mind that some patients, or those close to them, may have concerns that decisions not to attempt CPR might be influenced by poorly informed or unfounded assumptions about the impact of disability or advanced age on the patient's quality of life.

Conclusion

So how do I advise my trainees as they learn to manage resuscitation decisions and end of life situations? How do we allow doctors to apply their knowledge and experience of how treatments affect patients' function and at the same time discourage them from referring to such projections?

As usual it is all about the patient. We rely on patients to provide insights into their understanding of that projection. And if the patient cannot help us we turn to the families. Only the foolhardy march around the hospital making unilateral decisions about their patients' futures. But at some point it will become necessary to meld the medical insights that they can provide as doctors with the non-medical considerations that only patients or their loved ones can provide. Finding this balance is the real challenge.

The safest way forward will be to do everything, all the time, to preserve and lengthen life. For if it is true that we cannot be sure that even an extremely 'diminished' and inactive life does not bring rewards, then we must never be tempted to regard an image of the patient in the future requiring complete personal care and enjoying very little external interaction as without value. This must be balanced against a temptation to push our patients' bodies to the very limit. The danger in doing this is that we may condemn many people who are genuinely near the end of life to time that truly has no quality. Advising patients and relatives in these circumstances requires great experience, and although the evidence seems to show that we cannot hope to understand how they really feel, our understanding of how medicine, pathology and the mysterious process of recovery intersect is surely too valuable to be discarded entirely.

Acknowledgment: Lucy Series, who writes The Small Places blog, explored the David James and other, similar cases recently. Her insights were very valuable.

Deeper water: religion, end of life care and the case for public disclosure

We don't ask individual doctors about their religion – it is a personal matter. But religion and medicine are clearly interlinked, and this relationship is most apparent when decisions have to be made near the end of life. At this time religion can influence the expectations of patients and the management decisions of doctors. If a disparity exists between those two parties, and if the fundamental nature of belief does not allow one to accommodate to the other's preference, conflict can occur.

What patients believe is clearly important. The plight of Mr L, a Muslim man with hypoxic brain injury whom doctors did not wish to resuscitate in the event of deterioration, was brought before the Court of Protection in October 2012 by his family. They insisted that, based on his previous respect for Islamic law, he would have wanted every treatment possible that might extend his life. The judge found in favour of the medical team, Mr Justice Moylan saying,

> "It [resuscitation or aggressive organ support] would result in death being characterised by a series of harmful

interventions without any realistic prospect of such treatment producing any benefit."

Julian Savulescu (Uehiro Chair in Practical Ethics, University of Oxford), an atheist, has <u>written starkly</u> on the issue of unusual or futile treatment being offered in response to patients' religious preferences:

'Religion and ethics are different categories of human enquiry. Religion is as different from ethics as it is from mathematics. Religion is about faith; ethics is about reason. For ethics, religious values are just another set of values, to be treated in the same way as other relevantly similar values. Religion is about what biblical texts, traditions and figureheads say is right and wrong, and what some theists believe is right and wrong. Ethics is about what is right and wrong, about what we have reason to do, what we should do.'

However, my intention in this article is not to explore the infinite variety of belief that informs patient preference. We cannot reasonably expect patients to behave uniformly in matters spiritual, and questions of autonomy should not be invalidated by a religious background. Conversely, there is a school of thought that within a single health service patients should be able to expect consistency from their doctors when it comes to end of life care.

The questions that I would like to explore are:

i) Do doctors vary in their practise according to religiosity?

ii) Is such variety acceptable?

iii) If not, should doctors have to disclose their beliefs to patients? This question will lead me to ask, finally

iv) Should doctors disclose their beliefs in public debate on end of life issues?

Do doctors vary in their practise according to religiosity?

Clive Seale, now Professor of Sociology at Brunel University, conducted a survey of nearly 4000 doctors who care for dying patients. Having ascertained the type and strength of religious belief, he asked four questions, about the use deep sedation prior to death, attitudes to legalisation of assisted dying, the stated intent to hasten death, and willingness to discuss such decisions with patients. 13.4% described themselves as 'extremely' and 'very' religious, while 20.7% were 'extremely' and 'very' un-religious (with a bell curve type distribution in between).

Deep sedation was provided by 16.4% of very or extremely religious doctors compared to 22.7 of the strongly non-religious (p=0.03). Differences in intent (32.3 vs 50%), attitude to AD (anti – 15.5 vs pro – 51.1%) and discussion (64.1 vs 87.9%, p<0.0005 for all) were more emphatic. The headline result, reported in the media, was that non-religious doctors were '40% more likely to sedate than religious doctors' (<u>BBC, Today programme audio excerpt</u>).

The fact that religious doctors appeared less inclined to 'discuss end-of-life treatment option with their patients' was also highlighted, leading to conjecture that these individuals were perhaps complacent in their beliefs. A correspondent to the Journal of Medical Ethics, a practising Catholic, provided an intriguing explanation for this rather worrying observation:

"Perhaps the religious doctors only felt compelled to do so in cases when they felt the patient's suffering was particularly intolerable, whereas the threshold may have been slightly lower for non-religious doctors who have a more favourable opinion of treatment options that may shorten life. Thus, in the context of such extreme and apparently intolerable suffering, the doctors providing potentially life-shortening treatment may have felt that it was inappropriate (and even unethical) to delay treatment in order to engage in a discussion about this treatment option with their patients."

A tendency to shy away from full discussion of treatment options at the end of life was also found by <u>Curlin et al, in a 2007 NEJM paper</u>;

'Physicians who were male, those who were religious, and those who had personal objections to morally controversial clinical practices were less likely to report that doctors must disclose information about or refer patients for medical procedures to which the physician objected on moral grounds (multivariate odds ratios, 0.3 to 0.5).'

The Seale paper was not an isolated event. The Ethicatt study, published by Bulow et al this year, analysed responses by Protestant, Catholic and Jewish medical professionals in 142 intensive care units. It found that,

'religious respondents wanted more treatment and were more in favor of life prolongation, and they were less likely to want active euthanasia than those affiliated'

('affiliated' being nominal members of those religions, but without strong faith). A systematic review of the literature on this question (Mcormack et al, Palliative Medicine 2012) found that,

'degree of religiosity appeared as a statistically significant factor in influencing doctors' attitudes.'

Is this variability acceptable?
Following the press release and subsequent media coverage, a BMA spokesperson said,

'The religious beliefs of doctors should not be allowed influence objective, patient-centred decision-making...'

Was this a criticism of the state of affairs that Seale had revealed? If we assume that the spectrum of patient preference was equally distributed across the variously religious subsets of doctors who responded to the questionnaire, we must conclude that decisions were not being made on purely objective grounds. The preferences (if elicited), and the decisions that were made, were clearly modulated by the beliefs of the doctors.

Julian Savulescu wrote the following response to the question 'Should doctors feel able to practise according to their personal values and beliefs?',

'Objection by doctors, as is commonly practised, is discriminatory medicine. Only a fully justified and publicly accepted set of objective values results in ethical medicine as a proper public service with agreed and justified moral and legal standard to which doctors should be held.'

I have sympathy with this view, but think it is unobtainable, and possibly naïve. 'Is it right?' is probably the wrong question to ask. Variability is a fact of life, because all doctors are different and the practise of medicine cannot be completely protocolised. Medicine draws on human qualities from its practitioners, and the advice that each doctor gives is modulated by their own psychological and cultural make-up. We cannot expect or desire uniformity, for that would encourage doctors to perform at a remove from the very internal motivations that brought them to the vocation. That is why my third question,*should doctors disclose their beliefs to patients more readily*, may have greater relevance.

It is not wise to make blatantly religious statements to patients, nor to frame medical advice with religious references. The GMC recently found against a GP, Richard Scott, who, as reported in the Telegraph,

> *'told the patient he was not going to offer him any medical help, tests or advice and stated if he did not "turn towards Jesus then he would suffer for the rest of his life".'*

The GMC was accused on 'militant secularism' by Dr Peter Saunders of the Christian Medical Foundation. A case such as this takes us into rather extreme territory, and dwelling on it will polarise the discussion. Suffice to say, declaring ones religion in the wrong context is foolhardy. But should we expect doctors caring for patients at the end of their lives to mention, early on, that they have faith? To the individual patient such information would only be useful if that faith was definitely allied to a reluctance to prescribe deep sedation, or to take decisions with the intent of shortening life, or to enter into frank discussion. Would a religious doctor really accept that characterisation, or admit to such disinclination? I doubt it. That is the difficulty with large studies – it is almost impossible to know how they apply to the individual! So in answer to my third question I would to say no, it is unrealistic and unfair such face-to-face disclosure.

In the public arena however, my conclusion is very different.

Should doctors disclose their beliefs in public debate on end of life issues?

The Clive Seale paper is over two years old now, but I think it's findings, and those of related studies, deserve to be revisited in light of recent debate on the Liverpool Care Pathway (LCP), and in anticipation of Lord Falconer's upcoming Assisted Dying. Many people, from all walks of life, have been airing strong opinions. In these debates 'religiosity' is clearly relevant. Yet, while it is not routine for proponents or opponents to disclose their beliefs when engaging in argument, those who listen to their points will have little insight into the deep seated spiritual leanings that colour their statements. Seale concluded his paper with the comments, 'Greater acknowledgement of the relationship of doctors' values with clinical decision making is advocated'. *Acknowledgement* – that is the word.

The recent LCP controversy was sparked by a presentation from Professor Patrick Pullicino, a member of the Medical Ethics

Alliance, and was <u>followed by a statement</u> co-signed by a number of religious representatives. These included: Chairman of the Catholic Union of Great Britain, Chairman of the Joint Medico Ethical Committee Catholic Union, President of the Catholic Medical Association, a member of the Catholic Nurses Association, and the Founding Chairman of the Health and Medical Committee, Muslim Council of Britain. Yet these affiliations were not revealed, at least to the casual reader, from the outset.

It was only by looking beyond the newspaper reports that one was able to discover that the MEA is essentially an alliance of religious groups. This realisation led me to wonder if their arguments, which at first sight appeared to be based solely on matters of prognostic accuracy and patient safety (very reasonable concerns) were in fact informed by deep seated religious principles – such as 'sanctity of life'. The perception that life is God's gift may well conflict with a guideline that instruct the doctor to prescribe sedation which may, unintentionally, shorten a patient's life. I do not know this, because I do not believe in God, but it must be allowable to make conjectures linking the variations in behaviour revealed by Clive Seale with their possible psychological underpinnings.

If religion is driving much of the current argument about end of life care, we must ask ourselves to what extent these preoccupations can be allowed to influence national policy. For if policy is changed (or, more likely in the case of assisted dying, arrested in its evolution), those of us who do not believe in a God deserve to know how the care that we receive towards the end of our earth-bound lives has been shaped by religious belief. It should not be hidden from view, or made visible only to those who search beyond the surface.

Atheists must accept that religion is an integral part of life in the United Kingdom. We cannot disregard the historical events that led to the creation of the Church of England and its intimate relation to the state. Atheists must recognise too that much good in modern medicine derives from religion. Dame Cicely Saunders dedicated her life to the development of palliative care following a conversion from agnosticism to Christianity. Her obituary (Guardian, 2005) reads,

'Religion always played a part at St Christopher's [the hospice she created], though it was never forced on patients or staff: neither were necessarily Christian. The object was always as much secular as religious: to convince patients and their relatives and friends that they were not alone; that, despite their terminal condition, they still had value as human beings...'

As a result of the palliative care movement, and the way its associated philosophy has spread into the practise of general medicine, the UK's reputation for the care of dying patients is unsurpassed. The Economist Intelligence Unit found that the UK topped a worldwide 'good death guide' in 2010. Points were awarded for life expectancy, hospice availability and access to pain killers.

I am far more comfortable criticising religion than I am the religious. Who wouldn't be? All atheists number people with faith among their family, friends and colleagues. In this blog I have tried not to criticise, but to present evidence that belief alters behaviour, informs opinions, and shapes public debate. Debate in turn informs policy, and if those religious individuals and groups who take the initiative in the public arena are to maintain the trust of those who read and reflect on their views, I believe they should disclose their beliefs up-front, and not wait to be asked or discovered.

Notes:

References – I have embedded links to relevant references rather than produce a list here

Disclosure: I am an atheist

Part 8: The Liverpool Care Pathway controversy

Back to the source: a response to Patrick Pullicino's Liverpool Care Pathway paper

Why do this?

This paper, published by Professor Patrick Pullicino in the Catholic Medical Quaterly (Volume 62(4) November 2012, online journal), represents the intellectual foundation on which the current, frequently destructive debate about the LCP is based. The research into prediction, prognostication, treatment withdrawal and misapplication formed the basis of a lecture at the Royal Society of Medicine in July 2012. This meeting was convened by the Medical Ethics Alliance.

As a general physician, gastroenterologist and hepatologist I have been and always will be involved in the care of dying patients. Although I am not a palliative care specialist, and although I do not have detailed knowledge of the evidence for or against the LCP, I do feel that I am qualified to make this response. For I am one of thousands of doctors who have been accused, implicitly, of practising euthanasia.

I have not attempted to submit this critique to the Catholic Medical Quarterly as correspondence.

In this article I summarise each of the paper's section in turn and then present my own criticisms in italics. I have deliberately avoided trying to mount a full scale defence or overall justification for the LCP, choosing to limit myself to the points raised in Pullcino's paper. Excellent articles extolling the LCP have been published elsewhere. It may be helpful to open the original paper in a separate window while reading this.

Introduction

No comments.

Prediction and Prognostication

The difference between these two terms is discussed. Prediction represents an individual clinician's 'educated guess' of a patient's expected survival, whereas prognostication is based on objective data and statistical modelling. It is emphasised that data does not exist to allow accurate prognostication in the 'short term', ie. the 'final hours and days' for which the LCP is designed.

Seeking to highlight prognostic scores that address patients with very short term survival prospects, he describes the Palliative Prognostic Score. This study split patients into three groups according to their estimated survival, median duration being 76, 32 and 14 days. 30 day survival probability for the latter group was 17%. He then mentions a nomogram (by Felieu J et al, 2011) which gives a 15 day survival probability, but points out that it was inaccurate a third of the time. 'In this study, in a quartile (99 patients) of mean survival 10 days, over 10% survived much longer, with survival up to 200 days.'

These important observation force those of us who use the LCP to examine our thought processes. Are our prognostic/predictive skills really as bad as the literature would suggest? I know of no-one who uses prognostic scores and objective criteria on the ward. The diagnosis of 'dying' is indeed a subjective exercise, its accuracy increasing as patients display more and more typical clinical features. On further reflection however I concluded that the studies described are not particularly relevant to clinicians treating patients at the very end of their lives. What we are required to is recognise dying and manage it, not predict that dying will occur a week, two weeks or two months in the future. The question we must ask ourselves is 'do we diagnose dying accurately?', not 'are we good at determining how long this currently stable patient will survive with this illness?'

Literature search

The author states that no sources could be found to describe the use of prognostic scores within a 'very early time frame'

No comments   .

Clinical factors associated with withdrawal of care

This brief review concentrates on a study of organ support withdrawal in 15 intensive care units. It was found that subjective factors related to physicians' perception of survival probability, potential cognitive deficit and substituted judgment of the patients' view on resuscitation, but not age, prior functional status, illness severity or organ dysfunction were independently associated with the decision to withdraw. An accompanying editorial explored this phenomenon, raising concerns that physicians were 'creating a self fulfilling prophecy'; ie. deciding that death was inevitable and facilitating it's evolution.

The author then describes a study of patients with neurosurgical emergencies, reporting that survival was improved with aggressive surgical management and intensive care support. He concludes the section with 'Practitioners tend to be overly pessimistic in prognosticating outcome based upon data available at the time of presentation.'

Although a discussion about the power of physicians' opinions in end of life scenarios is valuable, and the danger of the 'self fulfilling prophecy' is of particular interest, I did not feel that

247

studies of ICU patients were relevant to the LCP. The vast majority of patients put on the LCP do not have organ support withdrawn.

Care of a patient put on LCP

A patient was admitted under the author's care and put on the LCP by a trainee in the context of apparently intractable seizures. Next day the author determined that the relatives were not in agreement with it. LCP was withdrawn. The patient was discharged and survived for three months at home with maximal support for activities of daily living.

The error here appears to have been a lack of communication. The LCP was not applied correctly, and the author's subsequent cancellation of it is not therefore surprising. The fact that the patient survived also demonstrates that the prediction, or prognostication, was inaccurate. My take on this case was that 'intractable seizures' is an unusual circumstance for the use of LCP, and the 'diagnosis of dying' all the more difficult. It is not surprising that the author was motivated to investigate the LCP following this experience. I wondered if the author's experience of LCP in a non-medical specialty had led to a skewed view of its benefits and risks.

Conclusions

The author states that there is no scientific evidence 'to support a diagnosis that the patient is in the last hours or days of life.' He then moves on to state that without an evidence base use of the LCP equates to an Assisted Death pathway. He highlights the very subjective decision making process, and recalls the problem of the self fulfilling prophecy.

The author then makes this hugely controversial statement: 'If we accept to use the LCP we accept that euthanasia is part of the standard way of dying in the NHS. The LCP is now associated with nearly a third of NHS deaths. Very likely many elderly patients who could live substantially longer are being killed by the LCP including patients with "terminal" cancer, as the above research shows. Factors like pressure of beds and difficulty with nursing confused or difficult-to-manage elderly patients cannot be excluded as biases towards initiating the LCP.'

The full import of this statement is explored below, but even if the accusation of euthanasia is overlooked, it must be emphasised that no evidence has been provided to support an overall rise in mortality since the LCP was introduced.

Other statements include:

'Starting a patient on the LCP, is an abandonment of evidence-based medicine in a critically-ill section of the hospital population'

Patients reaching the natural end of their lives are not critically ill.

'Nursing of elderly patients who are on the LCP in proximity to those in whom evidence-based medicine is determining care, is confusing to junior medical staff and nurses alike'

Although deserving of attention, there is no evidence for this.

'Use of the LCP is likely to have negative effects on elderly patients in particular, who are not on the LCP and to undermine the doctor-patient relationship'

This has certainly come to pass: trust between patients and doctors has been eroded during the LCP debate.

General critique

Defining prognosis and prediction is useful, although the difference between the two may seem rather semantic to many. As I have mentioned already, I am not sure that an analysis of our skill at prognostication is relevant to how we use LCP, the use of which is triggered by signs of possible dying. Nevertheless, if the LCP is perceived to guarantee death, it is very important that we identify dying patients accurately. Is this an achievable aim? Probably not. Should this admission result in abandonment of the LCP? Probably not. No methods of medical assessment, and no therapies, are 100% accurate or successful. As long as patients are reviewed regularly, to ensure comfort and to confirm the impression that the they are in fact dying, we should be able to minimise the risk of erroneous diagnosis while ensuring that the vast majority of patients benefit in terms of comfort.

It is the lack of evidence supporting the exercise of prognostication that drives this paper. The evidence that does exist in support of the benefit that patients derive from the LCP is not discussed. I think recognition that some evidence exists supporting the LCP would have added balance to this paper (for instance this 'cluster trial' – courtesy of Katherine Sleeman, Clinical Lecturer in palliative care, KCL, Cicely Saunders Institute).

Another area deserving discussion is that of communication. Prof Pullicino's paper touches on this only briefly, during his description of the man with seizures, and I wonder if a greater focus on family conversations would have increased its relevance in this regard.

My overriding objection to this paper centres on the use of the word euthanasia. It is suggested that widespread use of the LCP equates to institutionalised euthanasia, and implicit in this is an accusation that individual practitioners have killed their patients. To read this, as a doctor who has used the LCP, is very difficult. The accusation is made in the conclusion without any supporting evidence. The 'evidence' that is reviewed in the paper does not touch upon intentional killing. If we are regularly making inaccurate predictions (or prognoses), that is of course unacceptable and must be addressed, but the term euthanasia suggests that we are *intentionally* killing our patients. There is absolutely no evidence for this.

This paper, and the thoughts behind it, sparked a huge controversy over end of life care in this country. I think it is methodologically weak and structurally flawed. I think it contains baseless conclusions, and is excessively liberal with emotive, hurtful accusations of intentional killing.

Acknowledgment: Dr Rita Pal alerted me to the paper's online publication and has been helpful in researching details on the original RSM presentation.

Derailed: how the LCP controversy has changed family discussions

The Liverpool Care Pathway (LCP) debate has brought the public's attention to the possibility that patients are being deprived of life, their death hastened, when medical teams decide that their time has come. The elements of the pathway that were intended to reduce the burden of treatment, such as not inserting new intravenous lines or passing feeding tubes, have been portrayed as withdrawals of care.

The end result, at one level, has been helpful. Doctors and nurses are now more careful and explicit in describing what the pathway entails and what its effects might be. It is undeniable that in some cases, the LCP was started without families being aware of it. Most in the medical profession feel strongly that the LCP does not itself bring about death, but it has become necessary to consider this possibility when discussing it with relatives. But I now wonder whether this need for clarity has altered the tone of end of life care discussions adversely.

To put it simply, there is a danger that we end up discussing the philosophy and application of LCP itself more than the needs of the individual patient.

This may be because we are nervous. I can only speak for myself of course, but I have found myself introducing the term 'Liverpool Care Pathway' with a degree of hesitancy, because I know it may have baggage attached. I do not know how the relatives that face me will interpret those words, because I do not know how they have reacted to the media coverage. Will they assume that I am trying to enforce some form of euthanasia? Will they read into my words some malign motivation, the need to clear a bed, to unburden the Trust of their ailing loved one? Or will they have listened to the debates and read the articles without developing scepticism towards doctors? It is necessary to gauge the family's reaction before moving on to the next part of the discussion. And this carries with it the danger of the derailing the whole interaction. There is a danger that focus on the patients needs and previously expressed goals is lost, while the conversation segues into a cursory review of recent news stories and media reports.

You have no idea what the reaction will be until you mention it, but because the LCP is now 'controversial', you have to make emotional room and physical time to manage it. The tone is altered. If there is scepticism or fear (and who could blame a Daily Mail or Telegraph reader for having doubts after the numerous reports?) it remains for the doctors or nurses to overcome this, to gently persuade and reassure. Their skills and knowledge are diverted into justifying a mode of care that they continue to have faith in, rather than concentrating on the individual aspects of the patient's treatment.

One option would be to carry on regardless, to have the same discussion that one would have had before the controversy took fire. But that approach risks ignoring any concerns that the family might have but are too shocked or nervous to voice. There is a danger that a day or two later the import of the Pathway's initiation will sink in and the situation could be challenged. The bottom line is that permission is needed to start the pathway. Indeed, Jeremy Hunt (Secretary of State for Health) has suggested that it may become a legal requirement. This contrasts with resuscitation, which remains a 'medical' decision*.

So, what to most doctors and nurses was merely a way of organising and formalising established methods of terminal care has now become a 'treatment' in itself, one that demands a separate exploration of risks and benefits. I would question whether this is the right kind of conversation to be having with the family of the patient who is clearly dying. Is it really appropriate to introduce new ideas and new decisions at this moment? The medical journey has almost reached an end. The burdens and benefits of various therapies (chemotherapy, antibiotics, surgery, ventilators…) will have been discussed at length, but they will not have proved successful, and that is why the patient is now dying. As the patient moves into their final few days, the relatives are presented with yet another decision…one which, most believe, is not a true decision at all.

Critics of the LCP argue that doctors are not good at predicting death. This forms the foundation of Professor Pullicino's case against the Pathway. To a family member who has taken an interest in the controversy one of the first questions they might ask is, 'How can you be sure they are dying? I've read that it's a completely inexact science…' To the doctor or nurse who is trying to talk through end of life care options, this is hugely undermining. How can they introduce the concept of the LCP, designed to alleviate discomfort at the end of life, while simultaneously fielding doubts that are raised about the diagnosis of dying? The honest answer would be, 'We can never be a hundred percent certain sure…', while the unvoiced thought runs through their mind – 'I've seen hundreds of patients die, and I can tell you with a great deal of certainty, your mother is dying…'

Medical professionals can deal with all of this. Part of our role is to explain what is happening to families. We don't mind…but I do find it regretful that the very term LCP has become a potential stumbling block in a journey that should be smooth. Doctors, nurses and families should not have to be skirting around the issue of 'that death pathway they're always talking about…' when the minds of all involved should be focused on the needs of one person – the patient.

Note: this article is written with an emphasis on *non-capacitous* patients, rather than those who are able to engage in a full discussion before the terminal phase of their illness.

*best practice always involves explaining the resuscitation decision, and ideally obtaining agreement from the family. This occurs in the vast majority of circumstances.

An assault of trust: in defence of the patient-physician relationship at the end of life

The recent controversy about misuse of the Liverpool Care Pathway (LCP), arising from Professor Patrick Pullicino and channelled via the Daily Mail, has resulted in a sustained attack on the bond of trust between doctor and patient. It has been suggested that the LCP is commonly used to bring forward the death of patients for the purpose of vacating much-needed beds. The implicit suggestion is that very real economic and logistic problems faced by the NHS are influencing the therapeutic decisions being made by individual doctors. Critics of the LCP have been very emphatic and clear in their suspicions. Here are some quotes from Melanie Phillips in the Daily Mail:

In practice, however, the LCP has turned into something quite different. For while in some cases it has been used properly as intended, with numerous others it has become, instead, a backdoor form of euthanasia.

Horrifyingly, the LCP has become a self-fulfilling prophecy. When people are put on it, they are said to be dying. But they may not be dying at all — not, that is, until they are put on the 'pathway', whereupon they really do die as a result.

In other words, they are killed. What's more, they are killed in a most cruel and callous way through starvation or dehydration. And this in a health service that is supposed to be a national byword for compassion!

There are suspicions, based on much circumstantial evidence, that such patients are being dispatched via the LCP because — simply and crudely — the hospitals need their beds to meet overwhelming demand. This callous disregard for the most needy is of a piece with the all too frequent abuse of patients who are elderly, confused or difficult to manage and who may be treated in hospital with indifference, neglect or even cruelty.

Doctors who have used the LCP are therefore suspected of having killed patients and of bowing to managerial pressure to clear their beds. A direct, destructive link has been created between bed pressure and the purity of therapeutic contract. This requires more examination. I will now describe how consultants balance the pressures on their service and the needs of their individual patients. This is my view and I cannot speak for others.

The performance of doctors is under continuous scrutiny. Markers of quality are recorded and fed back to us on a regular basis. For patients the most visible aspects of quality are the efficacy of treatment, its safety, and the preservation of their comfort and dignity. It is difficult to measure these things, but patient questionnaires, the monitoring of adverse events and, with the help of outside agencies, adjusted mortality statistics, do provide useful information. Another important measure is the 'length of stay' (LOS). This is the amount of time a patient stays in hospital after presenting with an acute problem. It is accepted that the shorter the LOS the more efficient the medical system. Of course a short LOS is acceptable only if the patient is diagnosed accurately, gets better and has a reasonably comfortable and safe experience. But if we can be sure that our medicine is working, the next thing to concentrate on is its *efficiency*.

As more and more people reach their eighth and ninth decade of life, more emergency presentations occur. Having recovered from their illness many patients cannot go home because they have become weaker. In order to achieve discharge help from social services is required, for the provision of daily care at home, or placement in a residential or nursing home. This takes time. Beds are said, insensitively, to be 'blocked'. LOS trends upwards. New patients keep coming to casualty, but there are fewer beds in which to place them. Pressure! What do we do about it? How do we shorten LOS? Would I, would any doctor, really hasten a patient's death to this end?

What do I think when I see a patient who may be dying? My attention is narrowed. I perceive a man or woman in the last days or weeks of their life and reflect on everything that has gone before. It is an unscientific, almost poetic moment. I am privileged, in a way, to meet an individual at this defining moment. Everything that they have done, all that they have seen, resides in that darkening mind, memories betrayed by the frailty of the tissue that has formed them. I don't know them well, of course. I find out what sort of family they have, how many sons or daughters or grandchildren or great-grandchildren. Those family members may have already been to the ward and I, or members of my team, will have spoken to them. The details they provide form a rounded human being in the eyes of the doctors and nurses who barely three of four days ago had never heard of them. This rapid assimilation of impressions and emotions creates a three-dimensional image, albeit sometimes lifeless and uncommunicative, that is the centre of our decision-making.

As we consider whether to start the LCP we run through several mental processes. Is this really the end? Could a change in medication or management result in recovery and a successful discharge home? Would the patient wants us to work harder in an effort to avoid death or prolong life? Sometimes that the answer is obvious. Most experienced doctors will have seen over a hundred people reach the end of their life and the signs, although not scientifically verifiable or quantifiable, become recognisable. If it is obvious that death approaches despite our treatment we need to rationalise what we do to the patient. I have rehearsed some of these decisions in a previous blog post *('What we talk about when we talk about death: a case')*. What I don't think about is money.

Part of my role as a responsible member of the NHS is to use resources appropriately and efficiently. Sitting at my desk I frequently review my use of particularly expensive treatments or procedures, but on the ward in front of frail patients, I am a clinician. I am not naive – I do need to be aware of resources and make sensible decisions on a day to day basis. But death is different. A good death, if there is such a thing, demands care and focus. It doesn't cost much. Thoughts that do *not* enter my mind, as I look down on an emaciated, obtunded or cancer riddled patient, are bed management, targets, quality indicators or local health economics.

Yes, if the patient was to go home two days earlier, or to die two days earlier, the bed would be used by another patient, and a financial benefit could be calculated. My LOS data might look a little better. But for the clinician such a calculation is irrelevant. When a doctor meets a dying patient all such thoughts are banished. The bond between doctor and patient is at its strongest at this unique moment, and will not be eroded by such intangible concerns.

Paternalism at the end of life: a narrative from two angles

The Liverpool Care Pathway (LCP) debate has brought to the surface an ever-present concern that doctors have a tendency to make decisions unilaterally. The suspicion that important decisions are being made without the involvement of patients or relatives has led to accusations of paternalism and arrogance. My intention in this article is to show that this perception is, in some instances, mistaken. This is because behaviour may be interpreted incorrectly, and there may be insufficient understanding of the decision-making processes behind those apparently arbitrary behaviours.

A chain of events will be described from two points of view:

- a dying man's daughter

- a junior doctor involved in the decision to commence the patient on the LCP

First, we hear the relative's version.

"I knew my Dad had incurable cancer, we all did. He was two weeks out from his latest course of chemo when I heard from my brother that he had gone downhill. We went to see him and he looked awful, but he was talking, chatty even. And eating well. A bit yellow, which he hadn't had before.

"We called an ambulance and I stayed with him for seven hours while he was seen, going through A & E (quite quickly actually), then arriving on the admissions ward. He was given fluids and these really perked him up. The doctor said he might have developed some kidney damage, and the blood tests showed definite liver damage. But we knew about the secondaries in the liver...they had looked stable on the last scan though. I went home. Next day I went in after work to see him and he was on the same admissions ward.

"I didn't see the consultant in charge of that ward, it was very busy, but a cancer doctor we hadn't met before did come to see him, or so I heard. He cancelled the next chemo session which wasn't surprising. After that I don't know what happened. He was transferred to another ward that night. I rang the next morning to see how he was getting on, and the nurse on this new ward said he was worse, more yellow, more drowsy. She didn't talk about him dying. I said I would be in after work, and I got there by half-six but it took me another half an hour to find out where the new ward was. And he looked awful, really dehydrated. And more yellow.

"The nurse asked me if I had spoken to the doctor, and mentioned that the consultant had come round that morning. But no-one had called me. And there were no doctors on the ward, I think they'd gone home by then. I asked about the kidneys and she said they had got worse. The bag of fluid was gone, and I asked about that. The nurse said his cannula had come out accidentally, and because he was on the LCP they didn't want to put another one in. That's the first I heard of the LCP.

"That's why I'm complaining, no-one spoke to me about it. They just decided, on their own, these doctors who had never even met him before. They decided that it was time for him to die. He was supposed to have another two chemo sessions, we were still hopeful. The papers are right to bring this up, it's awful. He died the next day, early in the morning. I spent the whole night with him, they didn't mind on the ward…but he was asleep…I hope he could hear me."

The medical background

Mr Penny is known to have advanced bowel cancer with liver metastases, and despite ongoing chemotherapy has been admitted with a swollen abdomen and jaundice due to increasing burden of disease in the liver. Infection is quickly ruled out, but there is significant renal failure, likely due to dehydration. No other reversible causes for his deterioration can be found. The patient appears to have entered the final stage of his illness.

The medical admission unit team contact his oncologist, who agrees over the telephone that no further life prolonging treatments are possible. He offers to visit Mr Penny after his morning clinic, and documents in the notes that further chemotherapy is inadvisable. Although Mr Penny can hold a brief conversation it is not possible for him to engage in a detailed discussion.

Mr Penny has now arrived on a medical ward after one day on the medical admission unit. The time really has come to focus on his comfort and not be distracted by other treatments or interventions that will bring about no meaningful improvement. He has stopped eating, but does sip at tea now and again, and occasionally nibbles on biscuits. To receive enough nutrition for his bodily needs, from a calorific point of view, a tube would have to be inserted in his nose.

The junior doctor's narrative

The medical consultant responsible for the ward embarks on a ward round with his SHO (qualified for 18 months). They approach Mr Penny's bedside. He is thin, jaundiced and sleepy – semi-comatose in fact. As the consultant leans over he asks if Mr Penny can hear him. Mr Penny opens his eyes, meets the doctor's gaze and appears to focus, but after thirty seconds he drifts off again. Pressing on his abdomen the consultant feels an enlarged, knobbly liver beneath the layer of fluid.

266

"He's dying isn't he?" he says, having edged away to where the curtains separate the bays.

"That's what was handed over to me." says the SHO.

"Observations?"

"Stable actually."

"Do you know when the last CT scan was?"

"Two months. Stable disease then."

"Well it's not now. Has he been properly awake sister?"

"A few groans."

"He should be on the LCP shouldn't he?"

"I think so. He looks as though he's got a couple of days at most."

The SHO nods too. She hasn't seen many people die, but Mr Penny certainly looks close. All agree that the LCP is appropriate.

The consultant checks the drug chart and crosses out any irrelevant or unnecessary medication. These include a course of antibiotics for a chest infection that the admitting doctor thought he might have, but which was not confirmed on X-ray. There are also four cardiac tablets that were prescribed seven years ago when he had a heart attack. They will make no difference to him.

The consultant asks the nursing sister which family members have been seen on the ward. There is a daughter who attends when she can, usually later in the day. She is fully aware of her father's terminal condition but the nurse has no idea if she knows how close to death he is. It is arranged that the paperwork will be completed by the SHO after the ward round, but her consultant emphasises how important it is for the daughter to be informed. Then the small team moves onto the next patient.

At the end of the ward round the consultant leaves and the SHO examines her list of tasks. There are many of them…and it was made clear to her that the urgent clinical tasks should be prioritised. It takes her two hours to complete them. When she returns to the ward, after lunch, the nurse in charge gives her a fresh LCP document and asks her to complete the medical sections. She looks at those paragraphs that remind and require the medical team to check that the next of kin has been informed and are in agreement, but she cannot fill them out or tick those boxes because she has not yet spoken with the patient's daughter. Nevertheless she feels that it is important to complete the document because the decision has been made, and the care that her patient requires is encapsulated within it. She asks the nurse to contact the patient's daughter and request that she attend as soon as possible. A message comes back that the daughter will be arriving at 6:00 or 6:15. The SHO was planning to leave at 6:30, having committed to a Zumba class (she is aware of the juxtaposition, of the trivial and the grave, and accepts that she may miss it).

At 4:30 the SHO passes Mr Penny's bed and focuses on the task of communication again. Should she ring the daughter? She sits at the nurses' station, opens the notes and reads the home, work and mobile numbers. She lifts the phone, but hesitates. What if Mr Penny's daughter is in an office, with colleagues? Or in a meeting? What are the right words? She will be here in two hours, at the latest. Should you tell someone, over the phone, that their Dad is dying? She puts the phone down, and stares out the window, flummoxed. Her bleep goes off. Another patient, on another ward, has become unstable and it takes an hour to administer urgent treatment and transfer the patient to intensive care. This causes delays in all the other tasks and by 6:00 the SHO is well behind. The conversation with Mr Penny's daughter has been relegated.

The SHO arrives back on the ward until 6:30. She has tried to hand over some of the jobs to the doctor covering the evening shift. She cannot find someone else to have the conversation, for it requires someone who knows the patient well. It crosses her mind that the consultant could have offered, but he made it clear that he was in meeting at lunchtime and in clinic all afternoon; to be fair he did say he could speak with the family at ten o'clock next morning. Should she not complete the LCP? Mr Penny has been comfortable all afternoon and has required only one small injection of morphine for abdominal pain due to the swelling with his liver. The LCP is not needed for morphine to be given, its absence does not stop any palliative treatment. But the nurses keep asking for it to be done...that was the plan on the ward round, that is what is expected.

At 6:30 the junior doctor walks up the ward to see if the Mr Penny's daughter has arrived but the chairs around the bed are empty. She knows that the parking is terrible around the hospital. And then her bleep goes off again and she is called away. She never comes back to the ward. She leaves for home at 7:30 and in all honesty the arrival of her dying patient's daughter slips to the back of her busy mind. She hopes that when the daughter arrives a well-informed nurse will talk through the current situation. There were no indicators that the man would deteriorate quickly overnight. The necessary conversation can be had next day. It can wait.

Next day the junior arrives for work and suddenly remembers the importance of her mission. She walks past the nurses' station and heads to the end of the ward. She sees that the bed is empty. She asks the nurse what happened and sees that she has a grim expression.

"What happened?"

"He died early this morning, around 8:30. His daughter came in last night, you missed her I think, and she stayed all night."

"Was she OK?"

"No. She got quite distressed when she found he could hardly speak…and his breathing had become really shallow. She was present when he died at least, but looked really unhappy when she learnt that he was on Liverpool Care Pathway. Said the decision to do this had been taken without her consent or knowledge. I think she's going to complain."

[This is a fictional but illustrative case.]

'Challenge everything': a junior doctor questions the LCP

When a new junior trainee attended for his first clinical supervisor meeting I asked him to challenge what he saw on the ward, and not to be afraid to slow down the pace of things if he felt that his patients' needs were not being met. A week later he stopped the ward round to ask me why an improving patient was still on the Liverpool Care Pathway (LCP). In the ensuing discussion we pulled the LCP apart and put the pieces under a microscope.

The patient was 89 and had advanced dementia. She had been living in a residential home, requiring assistance with most daily activities, and was admitted following a fall with signs of a chest infection. There were also features of significant malnutrition. The home reported that she had been eating less and less there. Despite treatment with antibiotics and fluids for 5 days she deteriorated and stopped eating completely. When she tried to drink, liquid tended to tip into her windpipe and cause her to have further breathing problems. She could not cooperate with physiotherapists and the nurses stopped helping her into the bedside chair. She could no longer communicate, but appeared uncomfortable if she was not in bed. She just lay there. On one occasion her temperature was found to be 34.8 degrees C (markedly low), even though the infection had been treated. I decided that her dementia had progressed, and that she was now dying.

We discussed the LCP with her son and discovered that he knew all about it. He agreed that the time had come to concentrate on comfort. The paperwork was completed. Two days later, on the next consultant ward round, we found her sitting up, relatively alert, and able to tell us that she was hungry and thirsty. I thought carefully about whether to take her off the LCP but decided that she should remain on it, with daily review. The speech and language therapist was still concerned that should she drink there was a risk her lungs would be contaminated, but I asked the nurses to give her thickened fluids if she asked for them. The house officer wrote in the LCP booklet, looked at me quizzically, and asked –

Why is she still on the LCP?

That is a very good question. It's not uncommon for patients to appear to rally after a few days, on no treatment, and it's a real challenge to know how to respond.

She seems to have improved. Shouldn't we treat actively again?

We have to ask ourselves – does this improvement represent a genuine reversal in her medical condition?

But she has improved.

She has rallied yes, but has her underlying condition actually reversed?

Well, she was moribund, but now she is talking.

But look at the amount she's eating and drinking. Close to zero. Not enough to sustain life. So, really, she is at the place she was a few days ago just before she became completely unresponsive.

But isn't there a chance of further improvement?

We can't expect her to become better than she was after her infection was treated. At the moment she is alert but she cannot eat or drink enough to sustain life. So we have two ask ourselves what we would achieve for her by escalating her care again. If we put a drip back up to give her enough fluid to survive, what are we expecting her to do?

Couldn't we could try to get her back to the home, after a few days of building her up?

But we know that whatever we do she is unlikely to ever be able to eat or drink enough to survive in the medium term. It is her dementia that is doing that, and her dementia is truly irreversible. Should we feed her artificially? Well, if we give her extra fluid now, or a nasogastric feeding tube, we will sustain her life for as long as we choose to continue those treatments. But at some point we are going to have to withdraw those treatments.

Why?

Because it is not possible to send a patient with such severe dementia home on an intravenous drip or with a feeding tube in place. A drip means you have to be in hospital. A feeding tube is positively dangerous if you are confused and don't understand why you have it…which she wouldn't.

What about a PEG tube? [a feeding tube inserted directly into the stomach]

That is a good question, but we know from large studies that even inserting a PEG tube and guaranteeing sufficient food intake does not extend life or stop things like bedsores or infections. It seems counterintuitive but it is true.

But I don't understand how we can ignore her improvement.

I know it's difficult. But I feel that even though she appears to have improved her prognosis has not changed. She truly has end stage dementia and although the signs of dying that we saw a few days ago do not seem to have evolved, the situation is essentially unchanged. She is still a lady with advanced dementia who cannot take enough sustenance to survive.

So you think she is still dying, even though she…has improved?

I do, although perhaps not in the time frame that we anticipated. But if we now reverse our decision, put a cannula in, or a feeding tube, we will undoubtedly lengthen her life, but we will not change anything fundamentally. So now we have two make sure that her family are prepared for it, and do not challenge our perception that she is truly at the end of her life.

So while we do that shouldn't we take her off the pathway – shouldn't we make the assumption that life should be preserved? Isn't that our primary role?

I did think about that…about taking her off it while we discussed with the family. But is it right to chop and change if this improvement is really only a temporary thing? We must have the courage of our convictions when it comes to the diagnosis that we have made. You are responding to the evidence that she is now more alert, and assuming that this represents a genuine improvement in her medical condition. I on the other hand still feel that she is in the terminal stage of her dementia. Now you could accuse me of forcing fate by continuing to withhold hydration or food because in that way her ultimate death is almost guaranteed. I understand that point of view. It is an accusation commonly levelled at doctors who use the LCP. I would counter that by saying that if we now reverse our policy, we will be able to keep her alive in the short term, but it will be an artificial situation. It will be entirely dependent on the fluids (or tube feed) that we are giving. But then, at some point, we need to think about the next step. Staying in hospital forever is not an option. So be it her home or a nursing home, she will not be able to take in enough food or drink. As soon as she leaves here she will become dehydrated, and will begin to die again. So the life that we maintain here with our invasive treatments is not a fair reflection of her ability to survive. And it cannot go on forever.

So it's up to us to decide when she can die?

Perhaps. It is up to us to recognise when her dementia has advanced so far that it is incompatible with survival. It is our job, before that, to ensure that there is nothing more acute going on – like an infection – which can be reversed. And once we have ruled out or treated reversible causes we need to be honest with ourselves, with the family, and with the patient - if they are able to understand us. We need to be clear that she has entered a terminal phase. Is it not better to accept that and discuss it openly and make arrangements for a comfortable death, or for some time at home with community palliative care, rather than maintain her life artificially and hold out for some more fundamental improvement that we know will not take place.

But sometimes we are wrong.

We were wrong here. I thought she was going to die in the next day or two, and here she is engaging and talking. But I don't think I was wrong about recognising her still very poor short term prognosis.

And what if the family have the same reaction that I did and think that she should come off the pathway?

Then we have some explaining to do and some careful judgements to make. But at some point we have to test her ability to survive on her own, and it will then become clear. There are some other options. We should get a member of the palliative care team to give another opinion. And we should consider the option of discharging her off the LCP, and asking her GP to consider end of life care in the community if she deteriorates as we think she will. We review her tomorrow and if she has improved even more then of course, we will change tack. Are you happy? Do you agree?

I...

You're uncomfortable. That's good. If you become too comfortable around death you stop asking questions of yourself. I did ask you to challenge everything...you were right to.

[identifying details have been changed]